The CIVIL WAR HISTORY SERIES

INDIANA

IN THE CIVIL WAR

DOCTORS, HOSPITALS, AND MEDICAL CARE

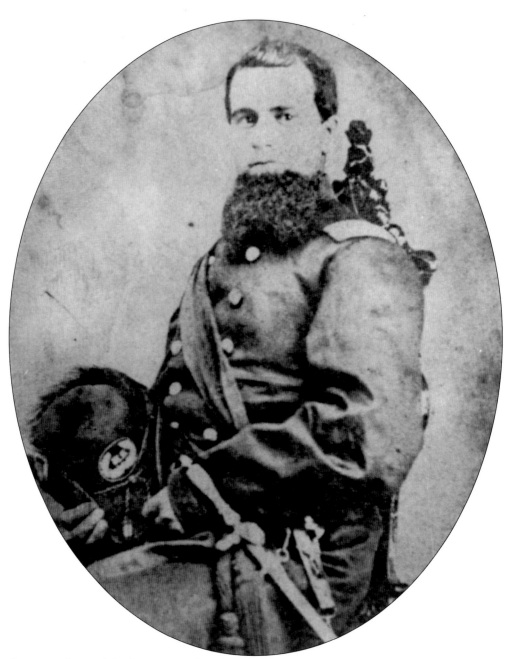

A new graduate of the University of Michigan in 1860, Samuel Pratt of Hebron, Indiana, was first an assistant surgeon of the 87th Indiana and later the 12th Indiana Cavalry. On September 1, 1864, near Brownsborough, Alabama, his horse slipped, fell, and crushed his right foot. (Courtesy of civilwarindiana.com)

Cover photo: This photo was probably taken at Aquia Creek shortly before Gettysburg. Present are officers of the 5th Indiana Cavalry. From left to right, they are Captain Torbell, Captain Farr (Provost Marshall), Lt. G.M. Gilchrist (in tent), Surgeon Elias Beck, Captain McBean, and Lieutenant Patton. (Courtesy of John Sickles)

THE CIVIL WAR HISTORY SERIES

INDIANA
IN THE CIVIL WAR
DOCTORS, HOSPITALS, AND MEDICAL CARE

NANCY PIPPEN ECKERMAN

ARCADIA
PUBLISHING

Published by Arcadia Publishing
Charleston, South Carolina

Printed in the United States of America

Library of Congress Catalog Card Number: 2001093326

For all general information contact Arcadia Publishing at:
Telephone 843-853-2070
Fax 843-853-0044
E-mail sales@arcadiapublishing.com
For customer service and orders:
Toll-Free 1-888-313-2665

Visit us on the Internet at www.arcadiapublishing.com

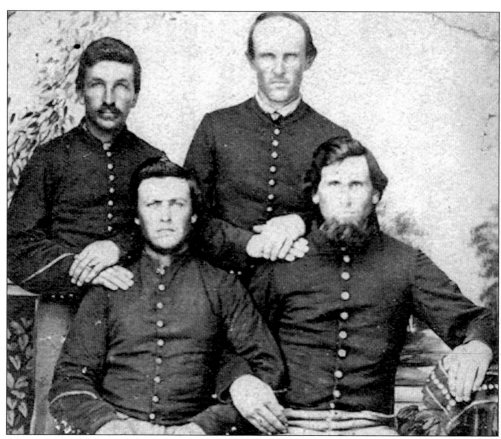

Pictured are members of the 8th Indiana Infantry. The 8th lost 166 enlisted men to disease and 84 were killed in battle. (Courtesy of civilwarindiana.com)

CONTENTS

ACKNOWLEDGMENTS

Acknowledgements to my fellow librarians of Indiana University who awarded me an InULA Research Incentive Grant in 2000—it worked; the wonderful people at the Ruth Lilly Medical Library for putting up with my writing schedule and all those past and present who contributed to my research; the collectors, John Sickles, Mark Weldon, Richard Wyatt Brown, John Croff, Don Wisnoski, Patrick Shcroeder, and civilwarindiana.com, who allowed me to use photographs from their collections; the staff of the United States Army Military History Institute; the Jefferson County Historical Society, especially Ron Grimes; Eastern Kentucky University Special Collections; Union University Archives; LaPorte County Historical Society Museum, especially Susie Richter; the Northern Indiana Center for History, Archives; the National Museum of Civil War Medicine; Peter J. D'Onofrio, without whose presence in reenacting I might never have become interested in Civil War surgeons; James Lee Berkley, who shared his photo of Cousin Ormond Hupp with me; Geneva McKenzie, who scoured South Bend and Mishawaka with camera at the ready; a real Southern gentleman and the expert on Indiana Civil War hospitals, Ralph Gordon, M.D.; and lastly, my daughter.

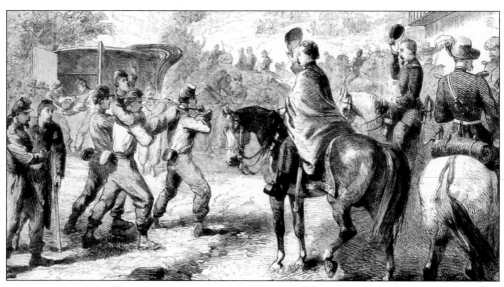

INTRODUCTION

Indiana's role in the Civil War was much more than the Iron Brigade, the Battle of Gettysburg, and Morgan's Raid into Indiana. Indiana contributed large numbers of troops who fought from Missouri to Virginia and Kentucky to Southern Texas. Several times during the war, Hoosiers at home feared Confederate invasion from across the Ohio River. Governor Oliver P. Morton was extremely involved in national policies and decision-making.

Civil War surgeons are remembered as drunk and always bloody. Writers of general histories of the Civil War include surgeons only as gory curiosities. Little or nothing is reported of their sacrifices and labors with the ill.

The Civil War battlefields in Kentucky and Tennessee are a day's drive from Indiana. Sites in Maryland, Pennsylvania, and Virginia are better known. Indiana soldiers fell ill in LaPorte, Indianapolis, Terre Haute, New Albany, Madison, Jeffersonville, Evansville, and other Indiana towns. Baton Rouge, Louisiana; Annapolis, Maryland; City Point, Virginia; Memphis, Knoxville, and Nashville, Tennessee; Louisville, Columbus, Paducah, Richmond, Bowling Green, and Cumberland Gap, Kentucky; and countless small towns in Mississippi, Alabama, Georgia, and the Carolinas saw Hoosiers fighting for their flag.

Indiana physicians were not required to pass an examination or have a diploma to become regimental surgeons. At the time of the Civil War, many physicians received their training as an apprentice to a more experienced doctor. It was up to the individual doctor to expand and maintain his medical knowledge and skills. Governor Morton took extensive steps to make sure Indiana troops were receiving the best medical care. He sent parties of surgeons and nurses to battlefields until the United States Army Medical Department was so well organized that no extra help was needed. Morton appointed nurses on his own, independent of Dorothea Dix and the eastern organizations.

Indiana had its own Sanitary Commission independent of the other sanitary commissions, such as the United States Sanitary Commission or the Western Sanitary Commission. These sanitary commissions were volunteer groups similar to the Red Cross. They supplied individual soldiers, regiments, and hospitals with supplies such as bedding, hospital clothes, bandages, special foods, stationary, and books. The United States Christian Commission also worked with troops in the field. Much was made of the fact that Indiana felt it necessary to maintain its own sanitary commission, even though newspapers reveal Hoosiers frequently sent contributions to many other sanitary groups outside of Indiana. An additional interesting fact about the Indiana aid societies was that women did not always yield the leadership of the groups to men, as was the case in many eastern organizations.

Governor Morton also sent military agents to such cities as Nashville, New Orleans, Memphis, City Point, and Washington D.C. who kept track of Indiana soldiers in hospitals in those cities. These agents could inform soldiers' families as to the location of their hospitalized loved-ones and direct mail and packages. While these families often thought it necessary to visit their relatives in hospitals, they seldom realized the expense involved or the strictness of military rules.

The soldier patients were generally young men away from home for the first time. Hardly any had ever been inside a hospital. The impersonality of a general hospital in the army was guaranteed to stimulate complaints from those well enough to complain. Certainly there were dishonest doctors, nurses, and attendants who stole from the supplies meant for the soldiers. To defend the medical staff against these claims, Dorthea Dix explained in the press that nurses needed to keep up their energy and should consume some of the food sent to the hospital.

The necessary simplicity of the regimental hospital in the field kept a soldier in contact with his messmates. When the army was on the move, ailing soldiers were left behind or sent to the general hospitals.

Doctors during the Civil War had few effective measures to fight diseases. They could vaccinate for small pox, give opiates to relieve pain, and amputate shattered limbs. Unfortunately, even the best-educated physicians in 1861 did not know about germs and infections. Though many surgeons had the skill to perform life saving amputations, infections often killed the patients.

The drugs the doctors had to use were often poisonous. Calomel or mercurous chloride was the standard treatment for intestinal complaints. Typhoid fever struck the crowded and often unsanitary camps before the first battles. Measles ravaged farm boy recruits. Measles led to pneumonia. Young soldiers often struggled to survive multiple infections while their regimental surgeons cared for them without the necessary supplies to equip their field hospitals. Doctors realized that army food was not conducive to general health or fast recovery. Indiana citizens answered their fellow townsmen's appeals for supplies and food to army camps, sending everything from jams and preserves to pillows and dressing gowns.

When Hoosier soldiers faced battle, the carnage caused by the rifled muskets and cannons overwhelmed the existing medical organization of the army. The army struggled to meet the medical demands of war on such a large scale. Eventually the removal of the wounded from the battlefield became organized. The organization of all surgeons during a battle insured that the best were operating on the most serious cases.

Throughout the war, Hoosiers were part of a gigantic struggle against death. Their stories reveal heroism, endurance, and frailties.

Abbreviations for Illustration Sources

Miller's Photographic History of the Civil War (MPH)
Harper's Weekly (HW)
Our Army Nurses (OAN)
Medical History of Indiana by G.W.H. Kemper (K)
Ruth Lilly Medical Library, Indiana University School of Medicine (RLML)
United States Army Military History Institute (USAMHI)

One

DOCTORS

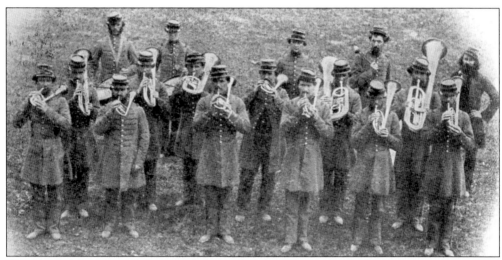

The 21st Indiana, or 1st Indiana Heavy Artillery, went to war with 17 musicians and a medical staff consisting of one surgeon and one assistant surgeon. A non-commissioned officer, called a hospital steward, completed the entire medical staff. All physicians commissioned by military units were called surgeons. The surgeon was in charge of all medical care, including morning sick call, and the hospitals during the battle. Assistant surgeons often did the battlefield duty. Stewards usually gave out medicine. At first surgeons cared only for soldiers of their regiments, leaving those with regiments held in reserve during a battle with little to do and others overwhelmed. Later in the war, surgeons were appointed to coordinate all medical personnel at the brigade, division, and corps levels. (MPH)

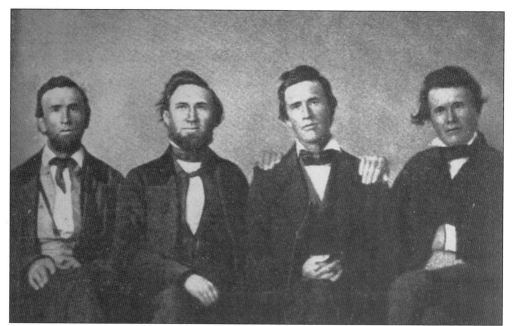

In this pre-Civil War photograph are pictured, from left to right: John Milton Wishard, Surgeon 5th Indiana Cavalry; Samuel Ellis Wishard; John Oliver Wishard; and William Henry Wishard, a special surgeon commissioned by Governor Oliver P. Morton. Joseph attended Wabash College for two years and then studied medicine with his brother, William. Later he attended Ohio Medical College and Indiana Medical College in 1877. He was captured during the war and was held in Libby Prison in Richmond, Virginia. (RLML)

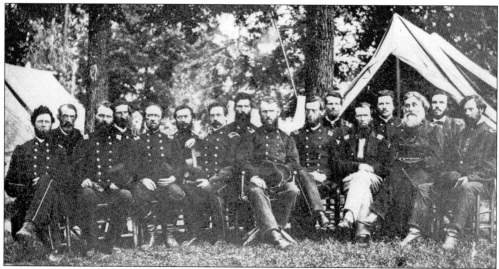

Sometimes in a matter of days, small town Indiana physicians such as the Wishards of Johnson County, Indiana, took on the role of military surgeon. Unaccustomed to the military and hospital administration, these men often found their best intentions blocked by military paperwork and officers with no military experience. This picture of the surgeons of the Army of the Cumberland contains several Indiana surgeons. (MPH)

"No reader of the Northern daily papers during the last year can be ignorant of the opinion generally entertained of army surgeons, and of the management of the medical department of the army. Inefficiency, gross carelessness, heartlessness, and dissipation are intimately associated in the mind of the Northern public with the medical officers of the army." So stated J.N. Beach, surgeon of the 40th Ohio Infantry. The photo is of John R. Robson, assistant surgeon of the 91st Indiana Infantry. (Courtesy of John Sickles)

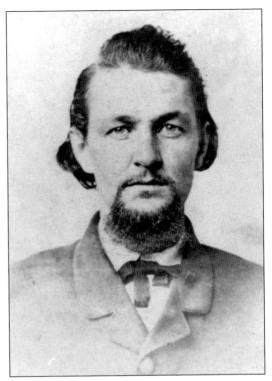

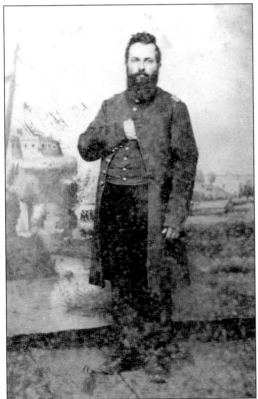

Dr. Beach continued, "During that time I have been associated with the medical officers of the troops in Eastern Kentucky, and Tennessee, I have met with but one drunken surgeon and few who were not making use of all means in their power to prevent disease and restore health. I have visited many hospitals where there was a lack of many things for the comfort of the sick, but none where the surgeons were careless or unkind." This photo is of John McChristie, of the 9th Indiana Cavalry. (Courtesy of John Sickles)

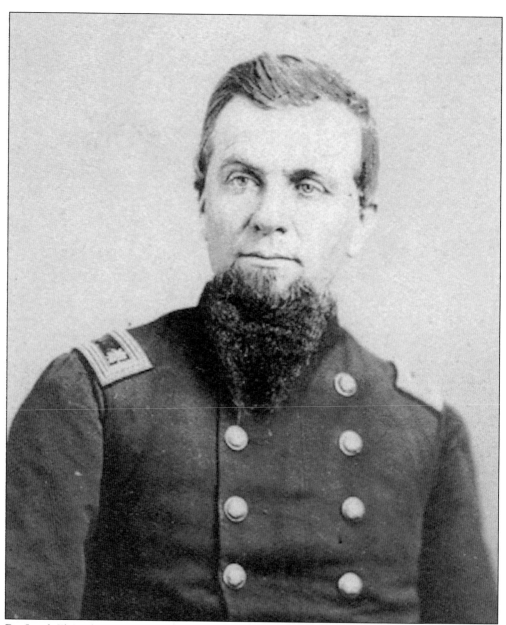

Dr. Jacob Ebersole of Aurora, Indiana, was the surgeon for the 19th Indiana (see page 22). He wrote, "The military surgeon's place and his work are of necessity removed, as far as possible, from the immediate place of danger and the actual scene of conflict. It is not his to plan the campaign, to lead the charge, or to inspire fainting hearts by deeds of personal valor, but faithfully, skillfully, and untiringly to minister to the sick, to attend to the wounded and comfort the dying. He understands what the soldier's life finally brings to many; the death wound, the burning fever, the wasted body, and the broken constitution. He knows what battle means; the shattered limbs, the moan of pain, the life-long cripple. Nor is his position devoid of exposure; oft times to personal danger, to privation, to protracted and exhaustive labors, while he is brought in almost daily contact with scenes and incidents of the most pathetic and touching character." (Courtesy of civilwarindiana.com)

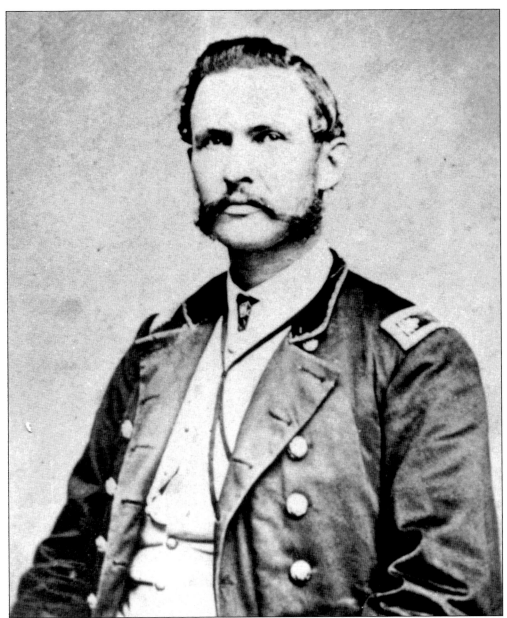

Dr. Ebersole continued, "The first and most important duty of the surgeon is to prevent disease; curing it is a secondary matter. The surgeon who prevents disease by a careful study of the causes operating to produce it, and who takes steps to remove these influences, is more deserving of credit than he who only thinks of curing. In the discharge of this duty it often becomes necessary to change the locality of the camp to make changes in the cooking and habits of the men to enforce what seems to them a rigid system of cleanliness of their persons, the tents and entire camp . . . and in doing these things we are frequently brought into unpleasant collision with our officers. It is not every military commander that understands the laws of hygiene, or who has the leisure or inclination to study them carefully; and the number is equally small who do not regard these surgeons who are always making changes and suggestions as troublesome at least." This is a photo of James S. Elliott of the 86th Indiana Infantry. (Courtesy of USAMHI)

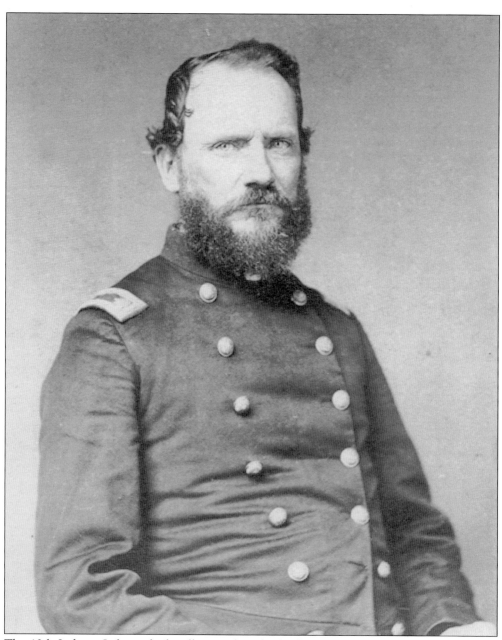

The 12th Indiana Infantry had well trained medical officers who served the duration of the war. Surgeon William Lomax of Marion, Indiana, is credited with having performed the first amputation in Marion using the flap method. Educated at Ohio Medical College and University of the City of New York, he founded the Grant County Medical Society and served as president of the Indiana State Medical Society. When the 12th went to Maryland, his wife, Sarah VandeVanter Lomax, accompanied him as nurse and matron of the regiment. She died of a fever in Sharpsville, Maryland, in December of 1861. At the disastrous Battle of Richmond, Kentucky, Surgeon Lomax had charge of the Mt. Zion Christian Church hospital. Later, Lomax became division surgeon, and in 1865, Medical Inspector of the 15th Army Corps at Goldsborough, North Carolina. (Courtesy of civilwarindiana.com)

Until 1862, volunteer regiments had one surgeon and one assistant surgeon. Later, a second assistant surgeon became part of each regiment. Alfred Taylor of Grant County served throughout the war as assistant to Lomax. In 1864, a member of the 12th wrote to his hometown newspaper from Grand Junction, Tennessee, "Our surgeon, Dr. Lomax, and his assistants Taylor and Campfield are all that we could wish for in the medical department." (Photo Courtesy of civilwarindiana.com)

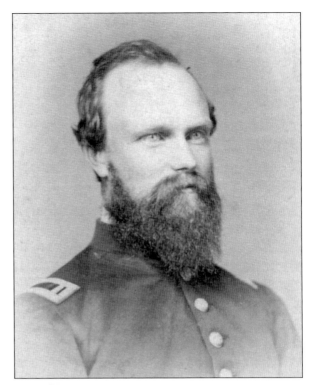

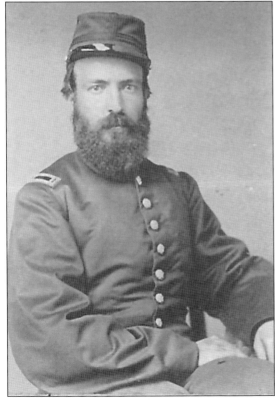

John A. Campfield enlisted in the 12th Indiana as a private, became hospital steward, and was later a second assistant surgeon. He was behind Rebel lines after the Battle of Richmond, Kentucky, and remained behind there for a month. A few months after the war, Campfield died as he was setting up a medical practice in Leesburg, Indiana, probably of a disease contracted during his army service. (Courtesy of Mark Weldon)

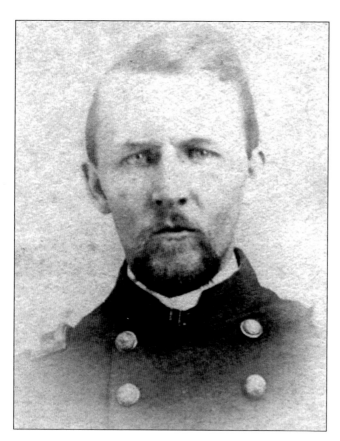

John Thomas Strong of Plainfield, Indiana, was surgeon of the 4th U.S. Colored Troops. Surgeons of African-American troops were white, as were the other officers of such regiments. When the regiments of African Americans were formed, many assistant surgeons of white troops took examinations to be surgeons of these new regiments. Medical statistics for the African-American regiments were tabulated separately from those white troops. There was an African-American hospital in New Albany, Indiana. (Courtesy of civilwarindiana.com)

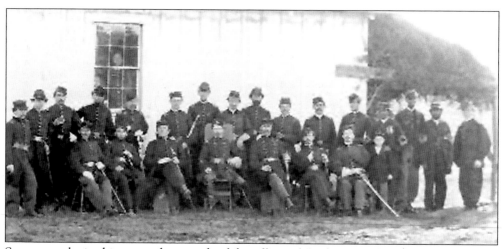

Strong may be in this group photograph of the officers the 4th U.S. African-American troops taken at Fort Slocum, east of Washington D.C. in 1865. Strong would have held the rank of major with the pay of a major of cavalry, but assistant surgeons were captains. In the regular army, surgeons had been captains and lieutenants. The pay of a major of cavalry was very attractive to many rural physicians, who seldom were paid on time or in cash. (Courtesy of the Library of Congress)

John Shaw Billings, the most famous Civil War surgeon with Indiana connections, was born in Allensville, Switzerland County, Indiana. After attending the Ohio College of Medicine and Surgery, he went to Washington D.C. for his examination to become a regular army doctor. Since he was from Indiana, many expected him to fail; Billings finished the exam with nearly the highest scores. (Courtesy of the National Library of Medicine)

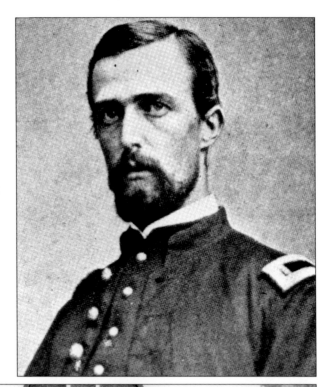

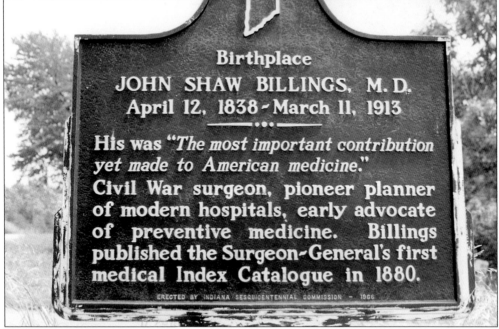

Birthplace
JOHN SHAW BILLINGS, M. D.
April 12, 1838 ~ March 11, 1913

His was *"The most important contribution yet made to American medicine."* Civil War surgeon, pioneer planner of modern hospitals, early advocate of preventive medicine. Billings published the Surgeon-General's first medical Index Catalogue in 1880.

ERECTED BY INDIANA SESQUICENTENNIAL COMMISSION - 1966

After the Civil War, Billings stayed in the army compiling important reports on the health of the army troops. In the Library of the Office of the Surgeon General, now the National Library of Medicine, Billings began the *Index Catalogue*, now the electronic index to medical literature, *Medline*, which is the cornerstone of medical research around the world. (Courtesy of J. Donald Hubbard)

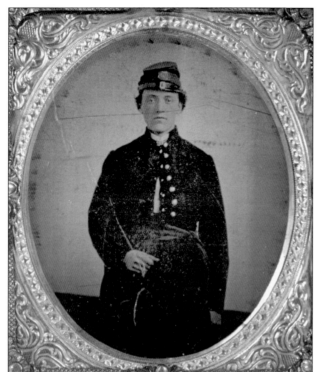

Hospital Stewards were the second highest-ranking non-commissioned officers in a regiment. They ordered the men of the regiment to take extremely foul tasting medicine. Often, stewards were trained physicians who enlisted as privates. James T. Jukes was hospital steward of the 57th Indiana Infantry. Jukes lived in the Philadelphia area at the time of his death, and there is no evidence he was medically trained. (Courtesy of civilwarindiana.com)

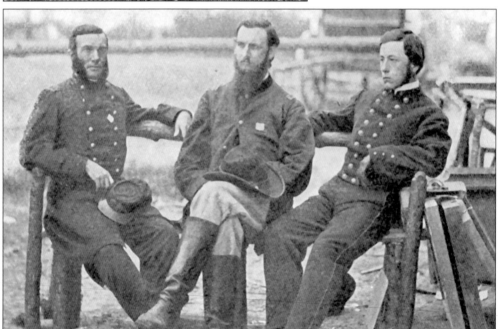

Dr. William R.D. Blackwood is pictured here with another surgeon and a medical cadet, on the far right. Medical cadets were part of the regular army "to act as dressers in the general hospitals and as ambulance attendants in the field, under the control and direction of the medical officers alone." Richard French Stone, a medical cadet of Bainbridge, Indiana, was a cousin of Confederate general John B. Hood (MPH)

William Commons was a surgeon in the volunteer navy. Since naval surgeons were not part of a state militia, they are not as often thought of as Indiana Civil War surgeons. An 1863 graduate of the Medical College of Ohio, Commons accepted a commission in the navy. William Foster was also a surgeon in the navy, and died in Texas. Philip Barton and George Beasley of Lafayette also served in the navy, as did Jacob Smith. (Photo Courtesy of the Ed Itala Collection at USAMHI)

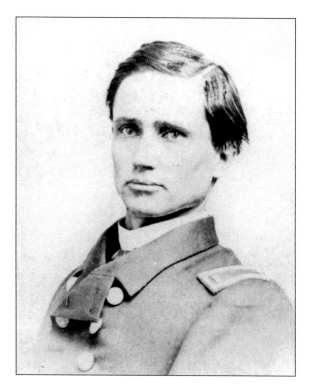

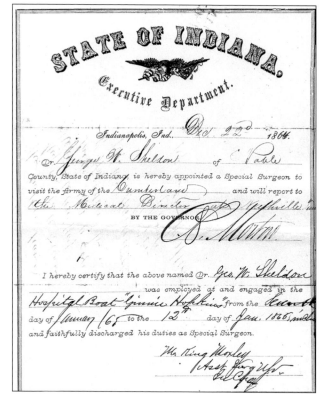

This was the "commission" received by George Sheldon, formerly of the 74th Indiana Infantry. Morton gave him instructions to report to the medical director of the Army of the Cumberland. His duty was a five-day trip on the hospital boat, *Ginnie Hopkins*. Morton issued orders to "special surgeons" whenever he felt Indiana troops stood in need of more medical care. Sheldon contracted gangrene while amputating at Perryville, Kentucky. (From the pension records of George Sheldon, National Archives)

19

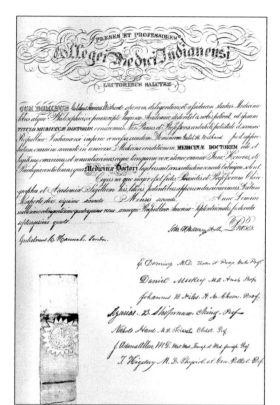

While regimental surgeons were not required to have diplomas, William H. Wishard did have one. Outside of Indiana, all Northern states had some examination procedure for surgeons. Unfortunately, examinations did not guarantee that efficient or knowledgeable surgeons would be commissioned. Many physicians who could pass the examination did not function well under the stresses of military life or were not strong enough to endure the hardships in the field. (RLML)

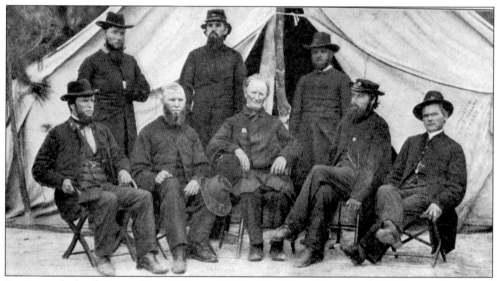

Regimental chaplains performed the multiple roles of nurse, postman, banker, and spiritual leader. Chaplains supplied necessary support to medical staff in the field and in the hospital. Religious reassurance was of great importance to many Civil War soldiers. Being spiritually prepared to die was critical to the well-being of the patient, his family, and his fellow soldiers. Many post-battle reports document the energy and concern of chaplains who worked along with medical personnel. (MPH)

Nathaniel Beachley of Bridgeport, Indiana, was a captain in the 26th Indiana Infantry and then an assistant surgeon of the 22nd. Later, he received a commission as assistant surgeon of the 69th. Officers described him as a temperate, energetic, and worthy officer, a gentleman at home and in the field. His colonel reported he was the only surgeon on the field from the entire brigade at Chattanooga, November 1863. (Courtesy of the Indiana State Library, Manuscripts Section, Picture Collection)

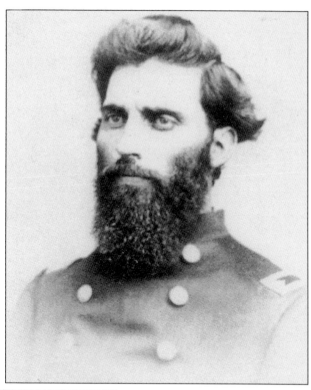

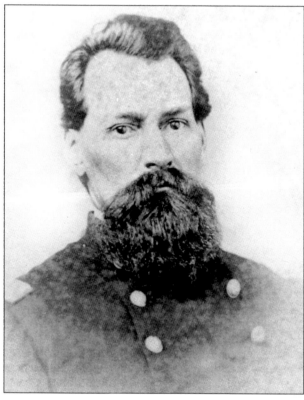

Richmond Welman, a captain in the 27th Indiana, was wounded at Winchester, Virginia, in 1862. He then resigned and was later commissioned surgeon of the 9th Cavalry. Many surgeons had more than one role during the war, working as volunteers and commissioned officers. Welman practiced for many years after the war in Jasper, Indiana, where he was a respected member of the community. (Courtesy of John Sickles)

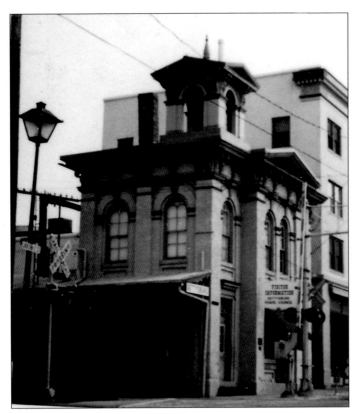

Dr. Jacob Ebersole of the 19th Indiana was placed in charge of a hospital at the train station at Gettysburg. He operated there for two weeks after the battle. Later, Ebersole received a letter from one of his patients whose leg he amputated complimenting him on the beautiful stump that was easily fitted for an artificial leg. (Photo by the author)

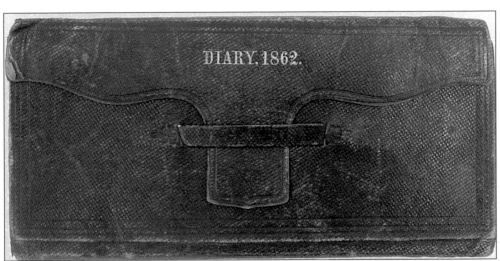

This is the diary of Jacob Ebersole of the 19th Indiana. Often the diaries of surgeons tell us more about what the volunteer doctors ate or how much money they spent than about their activities as physicians and surgeons. The official medical account of the war, *The Medical and Surgical History of the War of the Rebellion*, gives us numbers and illustrations but only hints at the drama. (Courtesy of the National Museum of Civil War Medicine)

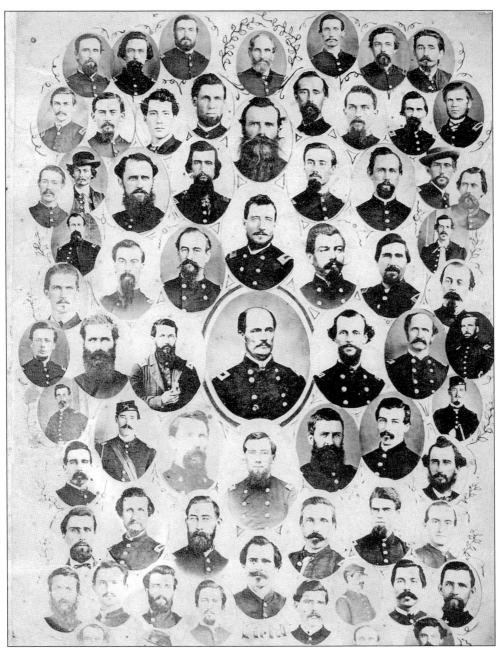

This composite photo of the officers of the 21st Indiana, also known as the 1st Heavy Artillery, contains images of not only the regimental surgeons but several physicians to be. In this composite is Captain Benjamin Rush Helms of Sullivan, Indiana, named for the physician who signed the Declaration of Independence. Helms would later study medicine with his father. Like Helms, some trained physicians who did not receive commissions enlisted as privates. Since physicians were often prominent members of their communities, they frequently raised companies and served as their captains. Some physicians chose to serve as line officers, feeling that this was more appropriate service as men than serving as physicians. Other men were inspired to take up the study of medicine by the example of the surgeons they met. (Courtesy of civilwarindiana.com)

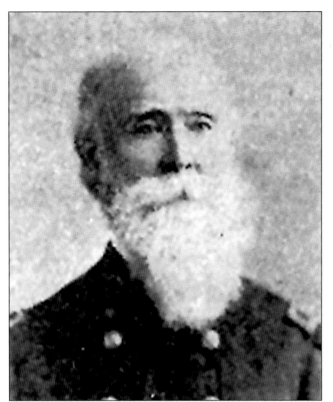

Charles McDougall of Indianapolis served in the Black Hawk Seminole War, attaining the rank of major in 1838. During the Mexican War he was stationed at West Point. He first served in the Civil War as medical director of the Army of Tennessee and in 1862 as medical director of General Grant's army and was made a brigadier general in 1865. He suggested a moveable hospital that could be towed from one place to another. The *D.A. January* was such a vessel. (RLML)

Livingston Dunlap was the founder of City Hospital, Dunlap's Folly. A letter signed "L.D." appeared in the Indianapolis *Sentential* in 1862, pleading that the nuns be supplied with daily transportation from the hospital to Indianapolis. "I can safely say that the greater part of the way to the hospital the mud is very deep." In response to this appeal, a wagon was supplied to the sisters at City Hospital. (RLML)

Two

HOSPITALS

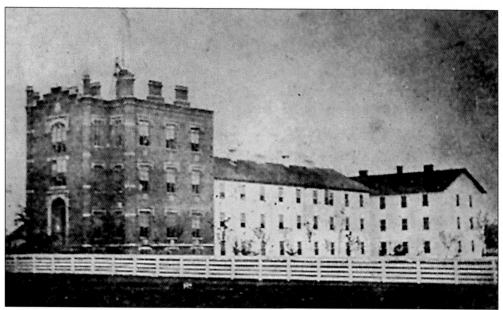

Indianapolis City Hospital, now Wishard Memorial Hospital, became a general hospital for the U.S. government in 1861. The wooden wing was added at that time. The Sisters of Providence from St. Mary's-of-the-Woods near Terre Haute took up residence as nurses. By 1862, the military hospitals at Indianapolis were so crowded with sick "secesh" that the old post office building was hired and fitted up with accommodations for 200. Fifty more patients were housed at the gymnasium hospital run by William Fletcher. Over the course of the war, City Hospital cared for 6,114 patients, including 847 prisoners. The father of a young man who died there complimented the Sisters for their unwearied exertions in behalf of the patients and added, "The efforts of our government to render, as comfortable as possible, our sick and wounded soldiers, entitles it to the gratitude of every loyal heart in the land." (RLML)

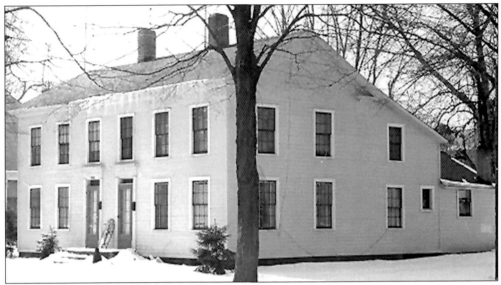

The training or mustering camps of Indiana Civil War regiments were located in each congressional district. Sickness, such as measles, mumps, and typhoid, quickly spread among the young soldiers before they even left the state. In LaPorte, Indiana, this house was a hospital for ailing members of the 9th Indiana Infantry. Although altered, it is on its original site. (Photo courtesy of the LaPorte County Historical Society Museum)

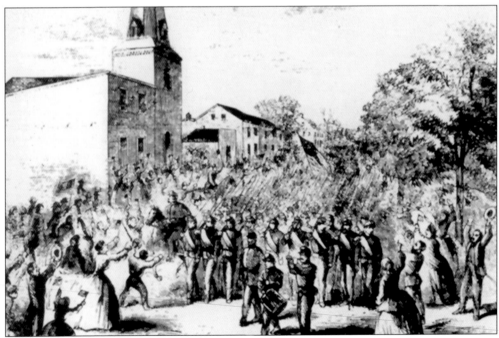

By the time the 9th Indiana marched into Danville, Kentucky, sick soldiers had been left in Indiana or would soon be in hospitals scattered around Kentucky. The physicians of the regiments realized that many recruits were not physically up to the demands of army life. Examination of soldiers before enlistment was at best haphazard. The fact that several Indiana women served undetected for months or years proved this. (HW)

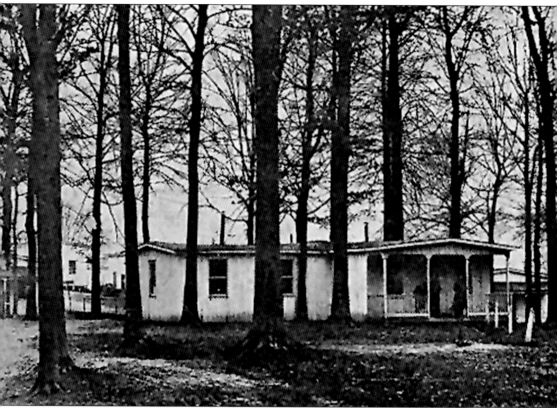

The general hospital at Madison did not feature a wheel spoke arrangement, as did the one at Jeffersonville. There were at least 55 wards or small buildings—each 125 feet in length, 25 feet wide, and 12 feet high, well lit and ventilated. Each building contained a stove, water closets, and a baggage room. Every tier of 11 wards had its own kitchen and dining hall. The facility accommodated 2,300 patients. The hospital also had a laundry and a stable. Surrounded by shaded lawns and a lovely fountain of cool, sparkling water, the physical facilities were complimented by competent ward masters, vigilant nurses, and good cooks with plenty of provisions. "All conspire to make the days and nights as easy and comfortable as possible for those within our hospital wards." (Courtesy of Jefferson County Historical Society)

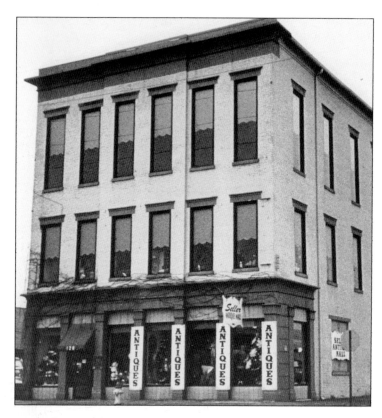

In February 1862, the *New Albany Daily Ledger* reported that the women of New Albany had procured buildings such as this for hospital buildings. The women also supplied the hospitals with equipment and supplies. The upper two floors of this building, one of which had been a ballroom, were used for hospital purposes. Not only did the women voluntarily perform this work, but they supplied most of the food and clothing for the soldier patients. (Courtesy of Dr. Ralph Gordon)

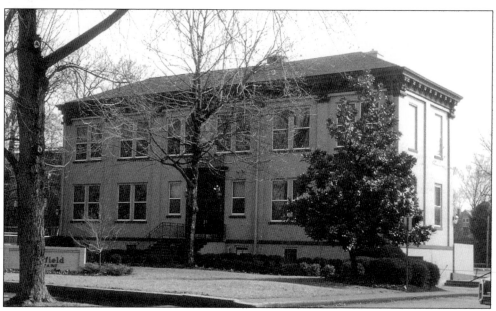

The newspaper in Madison, Indiana, reported that New Albany had offered to take care of 500 of the wounded at Fort Donelson. By 1863, most of the New Albany Schools had been pressed into service as hospitals. Many soldiers wrote wonderful letters thanking the women of New Albany for holiday parties including turkey, ice cream, and cake. (Courtesy of Dr. Ralph Gordon)

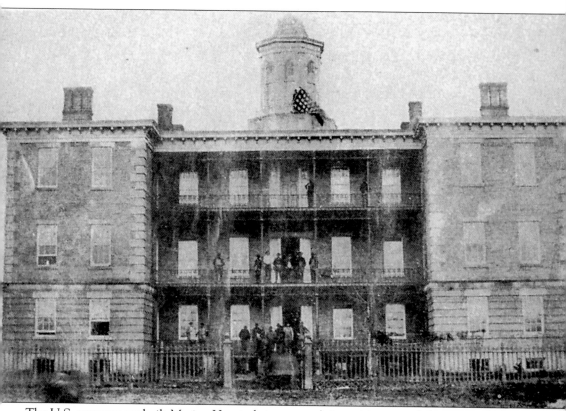

The U.S. government built Marine Hospitals in port and river cities around the country before the Civil War for seamen who fell ill away from home. The Evansville Marine Hospital and many other Marine Hospitals in several states were used during the Civil War as hospitals for soldiers. Robert Dale Owen's daughter served as a nurse in one of the several hospitals in Evansville. In December of 1862, R.C. Wood, Assistant Surgeon General, deemed the buildings of Evansville unsuitable for hospitals and moved 500 patients to Madison, Indiana. (MPH)

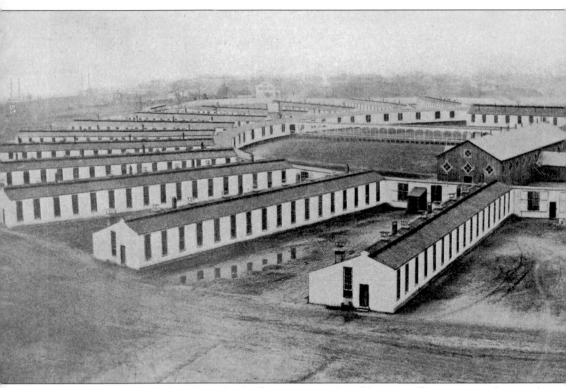

The makeshift hospitals with multiple floors were replaced by specially constructed general hospitals such as these in Jeffersonville, Indiana. At the end of each spoke or wing was a bath and water closet. The chapel and reading room were located in the barn-like structure in the center. The circular corridor allowed easy access for hospital workers to all wings. Hot water came from a central source. In the upper left of the picture is the Ohio River and a dock for the steamboats used to transport the sick and wounded from the battlefields of Tennessee, Mississippi, and Kentucky. (MPH)

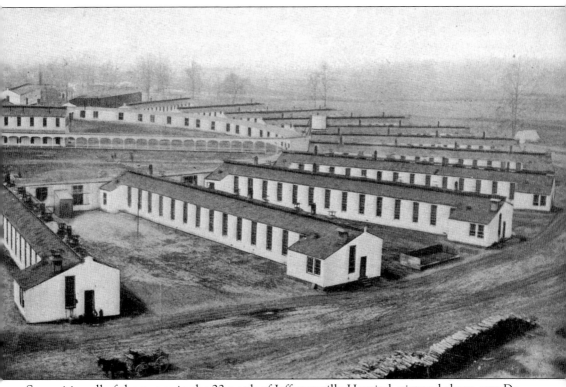

Supervising all of the nurses in the 22 wards of Jeffersonville Hospital, pictured above, was Dr. Cloe Annette Buckel. Some general hospitals in the East had their own bakeries and dairies. Although they delivered efficient service to the patients, the impersonality of these large hospitals was very strange to the soldier patients. In Indiana homes, the ill and dying were taken care of in the home by family members. Many physicians believed that the presence of relatives was considered important to the recovery of patients. (MPH)

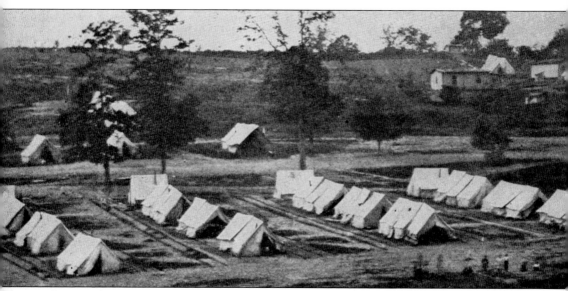

Camp Nelson, Kentucky, southwest of Richmond, Kentucky, was one of many convalescent hospitals that was necessary not only for those recovering from war wounds but also for soldiers recovering from such diseases as measles, typhoid fever, and pneumonia who needed long periods of rest. The need for these camps was unanticipated. The rigors of forced marches in bad weather and poor food made recovery slow. At first, soldiers were discharged and sent home. As military controls were imposed more uniformly, men were not discharged unless they were judged disabled for life. (MPH)

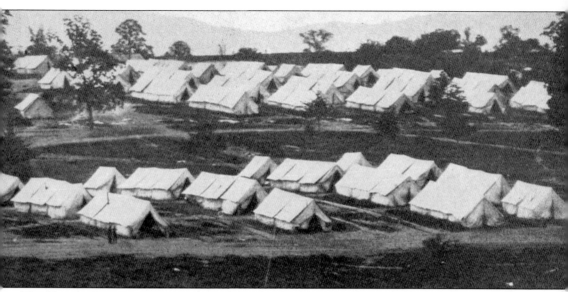

The Veteran Reserve Corps was formed for men healthy enough for clerical, nursing, or light guard duty. They had their own sky blue uniforms. Measles, mumps, and typhoid fever weakened men already stressed from long marches and poor food. Regimental surgeons were often assigned to these hospitals, leaving regiments in the field without any medical officer. Regulations were passed which ensured that a regiment would not be stripped of its surgeons. (MPH)

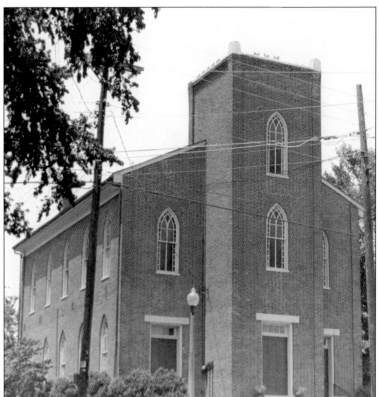

Presbyterian Church in Munfordville, Kentucky, served as a hospital after the Battle of Munfordville, also known as the Battle for the Bridge, in September of 1862. Munfordville was located on the north side of the Green River across from Bowling Green, Kentucky. Indiana troops guarded important railroads and bridges in Kentucky from attacking Confederate raiders. (Courtesy of Dr. Ralph Gordon)

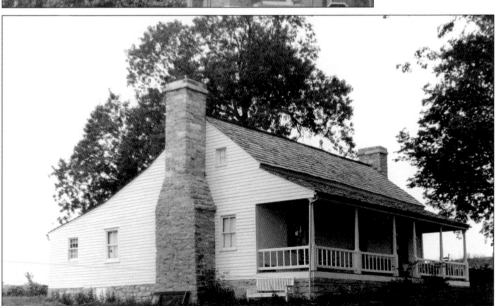

The Bottoms family house was on the Perryville battlefield in Kentucky. Ormond Hupp (see page 50) may have found shelter in a similar house. During the first years of the war there was no direction or organization for the removal of wounded from battlefields. Jonathan Letterman in the Army of the Potomac proposed a plan for the removal of the wounded and a system of hospitals which made the most efficient use of medical staff and resources. (Courtesy of Dr. Ralph Gordon)

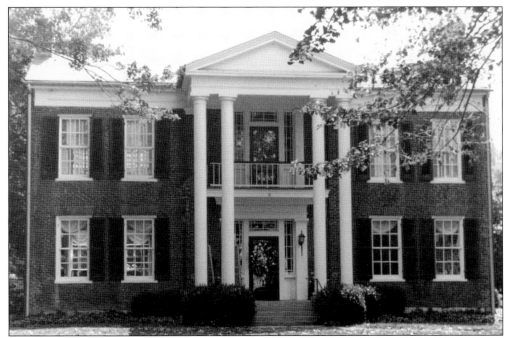

This building in Perryville, Kentucky, was used as a hospital after the Battle of Perryville. A court of inquiry at Vicksburg praised Union surgeons for preferring tent hospitals. Ventilation was thought to enhance health, especially with the invalid. (Courtesy of Dr. Ralph Gordon)

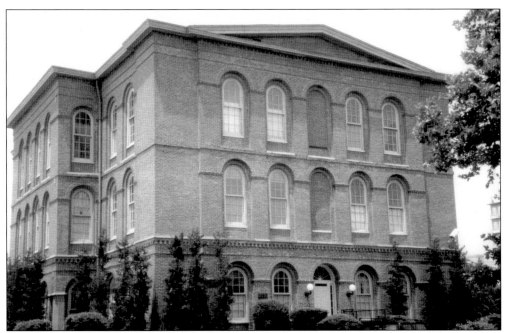

The Old Monsarrat School of Louisville served as Hospital No. 8 in Louisville, Kentucky. Louisville, had 20 hospitals in 1863 and 11 in 1864. Patients were transferred from Louisville hospitals to the hospitals in New Albany, Jeffersonville, and Madison. New Albany had a Hospital D'Afrique for African-American troops. (Courtesy of Ralph Gordon)

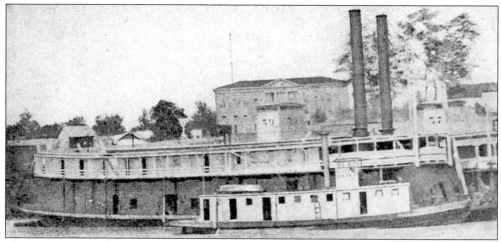

Mound City, Illinois, on the Ohio River near its confluence with the Mississippi was an ideal location for a Civil War hospital. A branch of the Central Illinois Railroad ran up to the city. Many visitors praised its cleanliness and good order, provided by the Sisters of Charity. A Hoosier from Kokomo wrote, "If God will forgive us for some hard things we have said about the Catholics we promise not to repeat them." (MPH)

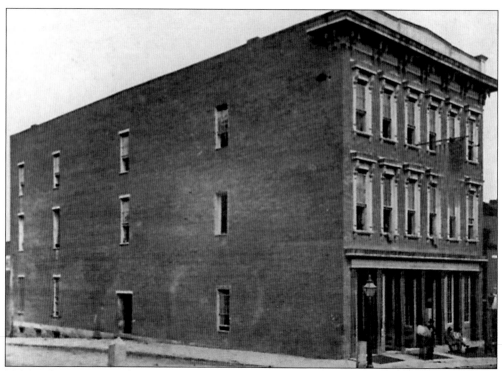

Milton Garrigus wrote home to the *Howard Tribune* of Kokomo from Hospital No. 19, the French Building at Clark and Market in Nashville, Tennessee. He complained that letters with money enclosed were often stolen by postal employees or hospital attendants. Citizens and soldiers were vaccinated for smallpox at this particular hospital. Passes were given to leave the hospital every day except Sunday. Garrigus experimented with phonography (shorthand based on the sound of words) while hospitalized. (Courtesy National Archives, J.A.H.)

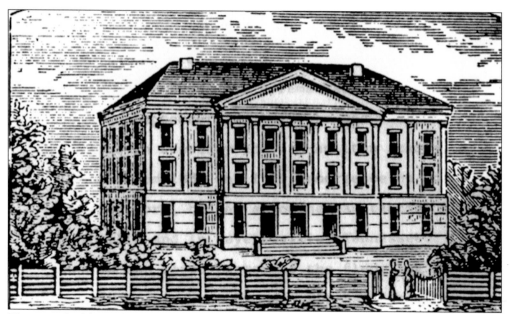

The main building of Union College in Murfreesboro served both sides as a hospital during the Civil War. Union University is now located in Jacksonville, Tennessee. Wesley King of the 75th Indiana wrote that the hospitals in Murfreesboro provided clean beds, rooms, kind surgeons, and the care from the kind ladies of Hoosierdom. He credited General Rosecrans and the Sanitary Commission with the excellent state of the hospitals. (Courtesy of the Union University Special Collections)

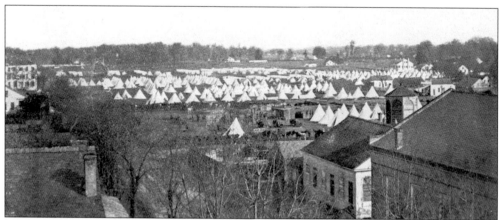

At Baton Rouge, Louisiana, in August 1862, federal troops from Maine, Vermont, Wisconsin, and Indiana suffered severely under General Thomas Williams. The general had tried to toughen the men with long drills and heavy knapsacks, as he had done in the regular army. His volunteers were suffering from malaria and dysentery. The prospect of battle got these men out of the hospitals and back on their feet when the general's discipline had not. (MPH)

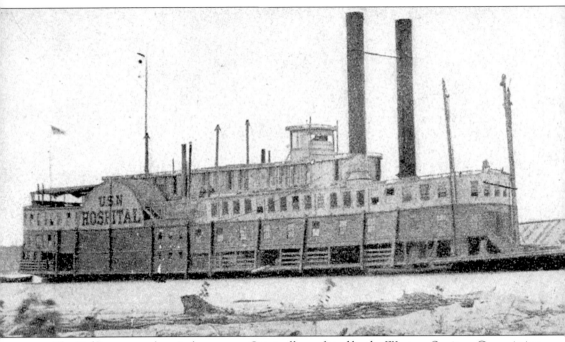

The *Red Rover* was a hospital transport. Originally outfitted by the Western Sanitary Commission, it later became the U.S. Navy's first hospital ship. Equipped with elevators, storage for 300 tons of ice, and gauze-covered windows, it was "one of the largest and most beautiful steamers on the river and has splendid accommodations for the sick." Aside from the amenities mentioned above, there were bathrooms, a laundry, an amputating room, and a corps of nurses, many from the Sisters of the Holy Cross as well as other female nurses. A crew of 47, plus 30 medical staff were provided. Such riverboats traveled the Ohio River from Vicksburg to Cincinnati. The Ohio, Mississippi, and Tennessee Rivers were natural routes for the transportation of wounded and sick soldiers. The army and navy provided no such transportation early in the war, so state governors and local volunteer groups had to charter boats and provide doctors and nurses to bring the wounded and sick back home. (MPH)

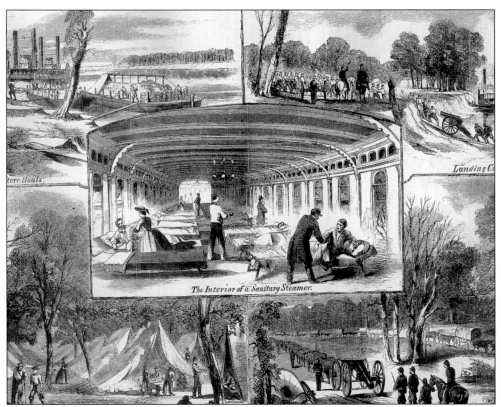

The Interior of a Sanitary Steamer.

The Battle of Shiloh was the first major testing of Indiana troops on the battlefield. It also proved the woeful inadequacy of the U.S. Army Medical Department in caring for the tremendous number of wounded. Riverboats sent by Governor Morton and other officials to carry the wounded from Shiloh caused a confused situation. Doctors nonetheless praised Governor Morton's quick action. Indiana boats would not take Ohio troops and vice versa. However, without these boats, no transportation for the wounded would have been provided. A husband and wife, Mr. and Mrs. A. Barth, were in charge of the hospital of the 40th Indiana Infantry in Indianapolis, and went to Shiloh to care for the wounded there. Many Indiana physicians went as volunteers to Shiloh on boats chartered by the governor. (HW)

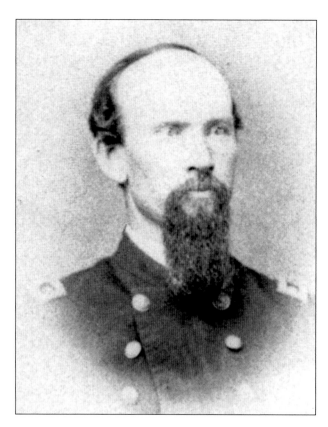

John B. Larkin, Assistant Surgeon of the 17th Indiana, was born in Vermont. He practiced medicine in Mitchell and Huron, Indiana. Detached from his regiment to the General Hospital in Bowling Green, Kentucky, Larkin resigned. He was re-commissioned in May 1863, while in the Officers' Hospital at Nashville, Tennessee, to Shelbyville to care for the wounded where he met his wife, Maggie Kincaid, the daughter of a local physician. (Courtesy of the Indiana State Library, Manuscripts Section, Picture Collection)

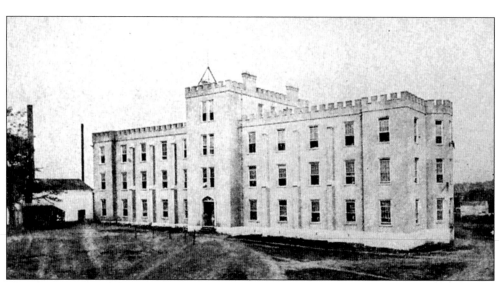

The Officers' Hospital at Nashville, Tennessee, was formerly called University of Nashville's Lindsley Hall. Officers were housed in different hospitals than enlisted men. This separation, though traditional in the regular army, must have seemed elitist to many Hoosier privates. Unlike Lindsey Hall above, buildings erected specifically as hospitals were always one floor, as to avoid patients having to be carried up several flights of stairs. (MPH)

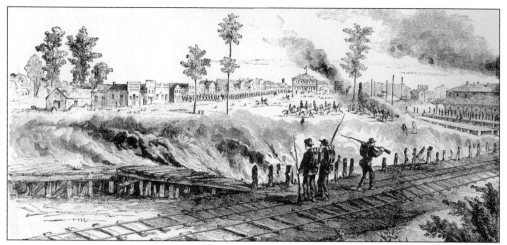

After the Battle of Shiloh, the Confederate army retreated to Corinth, Mississippi, and was held under siege by the pursuing Union army. Corinth was a new town and railroad center. Water was scarce for the civilian population. After the withdrawal of the Confederate forces, Union forces occupied the town. Already short on drinking water, the presence of an occupying army made water still more precious in Corinth, encouraging the spread of disease. (HW)

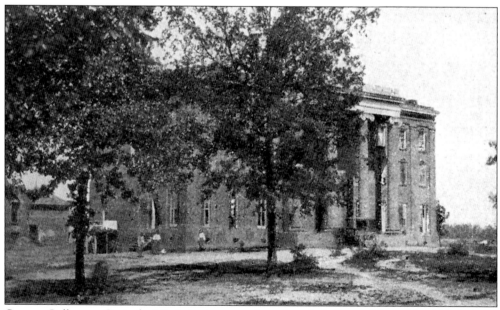

Corona College at Corinth, Mississippi, was used as a hospital. One soldier of the 66th Indiana wrote home from Corinth in March 1863, that there were 26 soldiers sick in the hospital and 43 sick in quarters. A month later, he reported the regiment was generally in good health—only about 12 or 15 in the hospital, and none of them dangerously ill. (MPH)

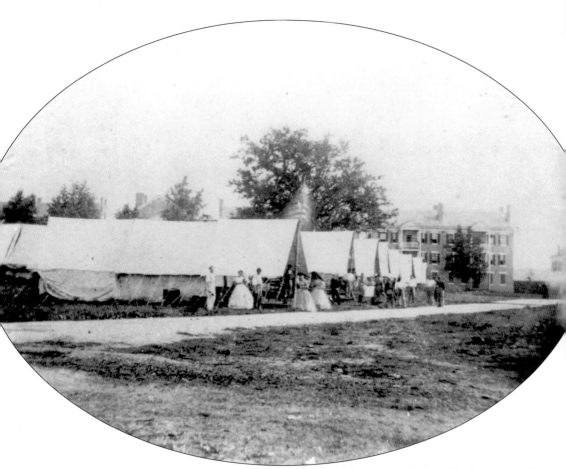

Mr. Rayburn went to Annapolis to see his son who had been wounded at Chickamauga. He wrote: "I visited the college hospitals and the next day went to the Navy Yard hospitals. The most pitiable sights I ever saw were here. They were wounded in every place imaginable, in the head, face, neck, arms, legs, feet, and body. Some were near starved—so near they could not tell their names before they died . . . When I came here I counted twenty-five three and two-story houses, fenced with brick walls on two sides, the bay surrounds the other two, with about one thousand men, every room, bed, patient, and nurses as clean as a parlor." (Courtesy of the Patrick Schroeder Collection at USAMHI.)

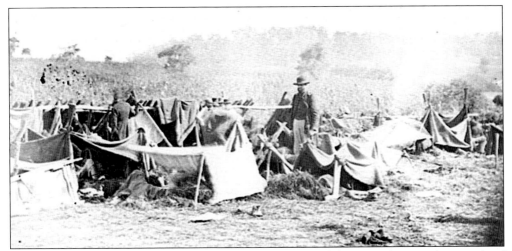

Anson Hurd of the 14th Indiana Infantry is the center of the most famous photograph of any Civil War surgeon. Taken at Antietam, the men in the makeshift tents are Confederate wounded. Surgeons cared for the wounded of either side. Although one female nurse reported she could not take care of Confederate patients, these were exceptions. (Courtesy of the Library of Congress)

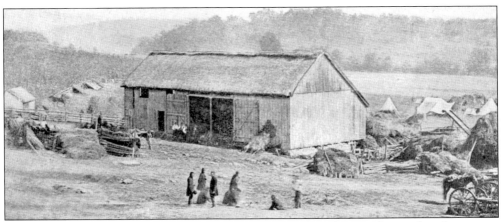

This barn at Antietam was used as a hospital. Barns were often chosen as hospitals and operating sites, as they offered the largest number of covered space in open countrysides, and generally near a water source. Unfortunately, while barns were convenient, they also harbored animal waste and other sources of infection. Better structures proved to be churches, since they were generally cleaner and provided pews that could serve as beds. (MPH)

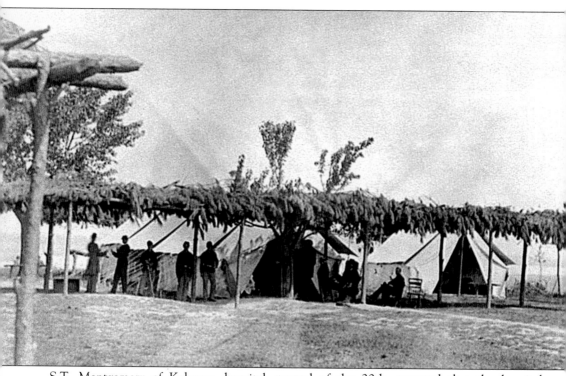

S.T. Montgomery of Kokomo, hospital steward of the 20th, reported that the hospital accommodations were excellent at City Point, Virginia. He called it the most complete depot for the sick and wounded and reported that the men were as well cared for there as at most of the fort hospitals. Tents there were arranged in rows along wide streets and were cooler in summer than buildings. In front of the canvas buildings were arbors of pine boughs. Each building was entered through arches made of spruce twigs, and each side of the street was lined with shade trees. The 2nd Corps alone had 10 to 12 acres. Montgomery worked in the dispensary with hospital stewards from Maine, Massachusetts, New Jersey, Pennsylvania, and Minnesota, and reported that they were men of talent and honor. (MPH)

Three

ILLNESS AND INJURY

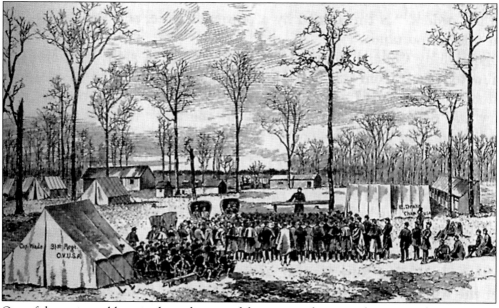

One of the main problems in the early years of the war was the proper location and construction of privies. The presence of horses added greatly to the probability that water would become contaminated. Training the men to make use of the privies was also a matter of great importance. In an era when surgeons did not wash their hands, it is not surprising that camps where six or more men shared a tent, diseases spread out of control. Immigrant soldiers who had already been exposed to typhoid on ships were often immune and were spared this deadly disease. As well, city regiments often suffered less from communicable disease because they had been exposed to more diseases within the larger cities. At Camp Dick Robinson located near Perryville and Bardstown, Kentucky, the men of an Ohio Regiment are listening to a sermon. (HW)

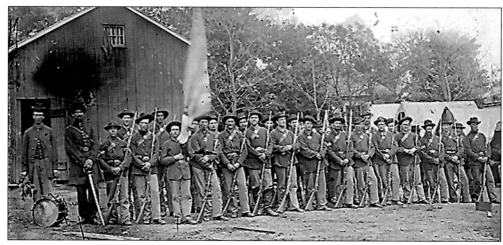

Regiments such as the 44th Indiana, pictured here, found that measles, typhoid fever, pneumonia, and dysentery were more frequent killers than enemy bullets. These diseases also struck civilians in Indiana, but for the soldier lacking rest and proper food, they were deadlier. "Comfortless sickness, disconsolate deathbeds, burials with the doleful wail of marital music and the presence of no weeping woman—these are the foremost recollections of the encampment at Nolin Creek, Kentucky," one Hoosier remembered. (MPH)

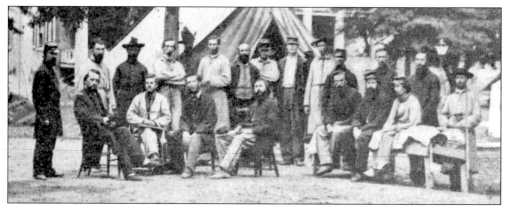

This photograph is of a small group of patients taken during the Red River Campaign in Lousiana. Several are dressed in hospital robes. Clothing for the sick and wounded was scarce on many campaigns. Access to water and soap was also limited. Surgeons had to rely on relief or sanitary commissions for their supplies of bedding, specialty foods, and often hospital clothing. (MPH)

Samuel Sawyer, chaplain of the 47th, described Dr. James L. Dicken's daily sick call: "At 6:30 in the morning he stands behind his board counter, and examines the patients sent to him from the different companies and excuses them from duty or not as he may deem proper. He then sends them to Dr. James, who administers remedies to suit the complaint." Dr. Dicken was from Wabash, Indiana. (RLML)

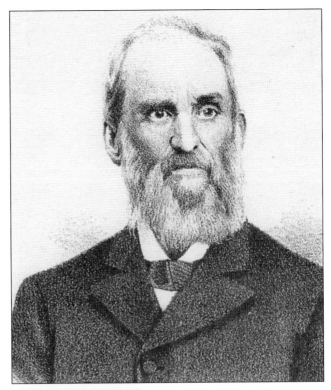

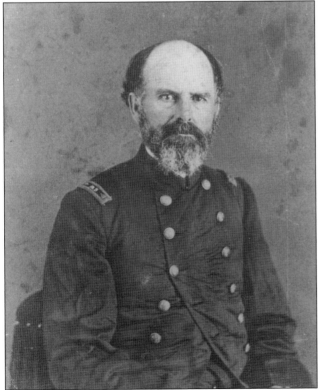

Joseph G. McPheeters of Bloomington, Indiana, attended Indiana University and Transylvania University's Medical Department. He served with the 14th for three months and was with the 33rd from 1861 until 1864. In August 1861, he wrote to the Terre Haute *Daily Express*, "During the last two weeks there has been an increase of disease in the regiment, occasioned by incessant rain, and damp quarters. No measles."(Courtesy of the William C. Ambrose Collection at USAMHI)

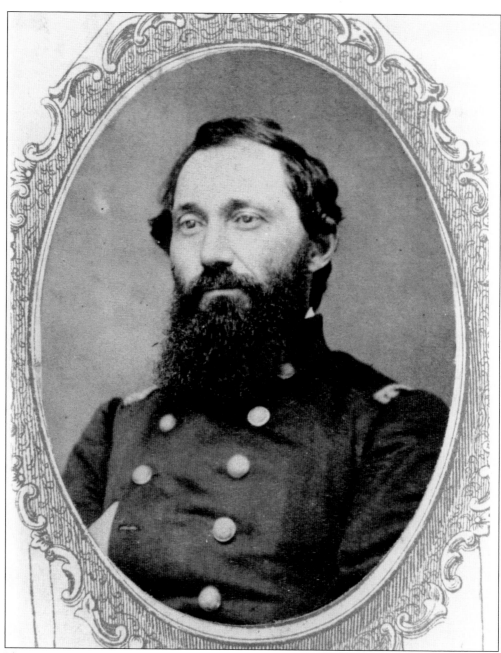

Elias W.H. Beck of the 3rd Indiana Cavalry, right wing, was prominent not only for his medical abilities but also for being the son-in-law of General Samuel Milroy, with whom he served as surgeon during the Mexican War. Beck wrote wonderful letters home to his wife Francis, who was a temperance crusader. Both Becks were interested in spiritualism. Influenced by his father-in-law's fame, he was constantly apologizing to his wife for his meager income as, "I am working for $6 a day cash, for to further the interests of my family." September 19, 1862, Beck wrote to his wife that he performed six amputations and would have more to do tomorrow. He was promoted to Brigade and Division Surgeon. In one of his letters from Aquia Creek, he mentions having his picture taken in camp. It may be the one on the cover of this book. (Courtesy of John Sickles)

Early in the war, the Surgeon General of the U.S. Army requested interesting cases and anatomical specimens be sent to his office. This photograph was taken when Bugler J.H. Ewing visited the Army Medical Museum in 1865. The statistics, cases, and reports after battles were compiled into the *Medical and Surgical History of the War of the Rebellion* (reprinted as *The Medical and Surgical History of the Civil War*). This multi-volume work was hailed as one of the greatest contributions to medicine made by Americans to that date. (MSHWR)

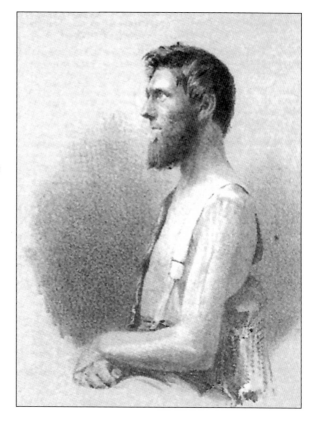

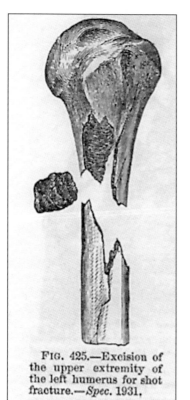

FIG. 425.—Excision of the upper extremity of the left humerus for shot fracture.—*Spec.* 1931.

This is an illustration of bone excised from the arm of Bugler J.H. Ewing, 8th Illinois Cavalry at Culpepper, November 8, 1863, by surgeon Elias Beck at the Cavalry Corps Hospital. Ewing suffered little blood loss. Although he would always suffer pain in the arm and it required a brace, he recovered some use it. If Ewing suffered pain, even part of the time, one wonders if the excision was preferable to amputation. (MSHWR)

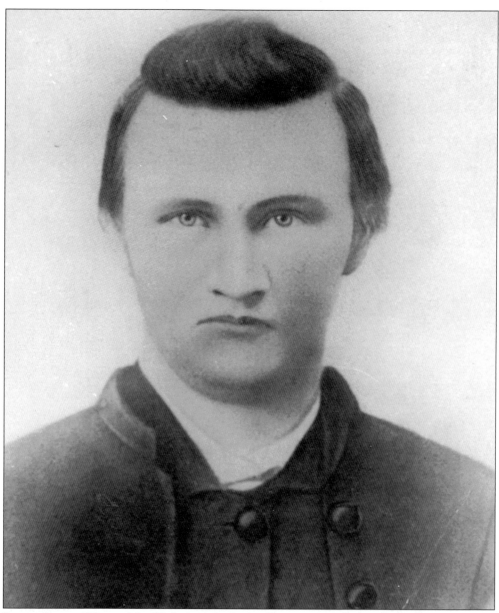

Private Ormond Hupp of the 5th Indiana Light Artillery was wounded at the Battle of Perryville. An ammunition chest blew up, tossing him 10 feet into the air and giving him painful but survivable powder burns. He walked to one field hospital where a surgeon wanted to take off his arm. Hupp left, believing correctly that the surgeon was frightened out his wits by the surrounding battle. Soon after, he came across a man passing out whiskey. He would have had too much if a fellow artillerist had not stopped him. Hupp's friend got him to a surgeon who dressed the wound and put "sweet oil" on his burns. He took shelter at a farm near his battery's position until his brigade ambulance picked him up. He made his way with many others to Louisville and then on to New Albany, Indiana. He worked as a nurse in the hospital for many months and made many friends among the women of New Albany. (Courtesy of John Lee Berkley)

Dr. John Sloan met Ormund Hupp on the dock in New Albany. A native of Maine and educated at Bowdoin College, his medical career spanned the age of bleedings to antiseptic surgery. He was originally the post surgeon at New Albany but the military soon sent in Dr. Thomas W. Fry of Crawfordsville to be in charge of the hospitals in that region. (RLML)

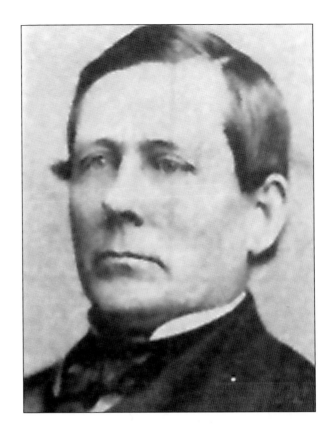

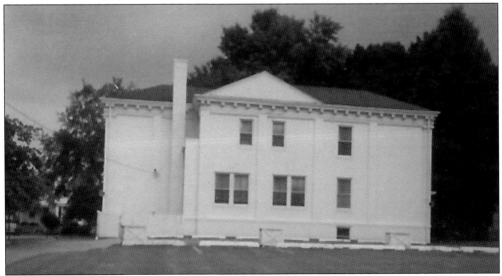

Early in the war the people of New Albany, Indiana, transformed their school buildings into hospitals. This building was Upper City School before it became Hospital No. 1. At one time, there were 11 hospitals scattered around the town. Although this was a unique volunteer effort, it was not efficient use of staff and space. New Albany competed with Louisville for assignment of patients. (Courtesy of John Lee Berkley)

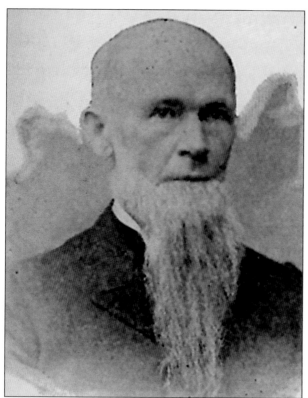

William Wylie Blair of Princeton, Indiana, was surgeon of the 58th Indiana Infantry. He reported during the Battle of Murfreesboro that there were three operating teams, consisting of a surgeon and three assistants. The remaining assistant surgeons, stewards, and experienced nurses dressed slighter wounds. He required stragglers to do police duty in the camp. He also reported that amputations were seldom performed without consultation. (Regimental History)

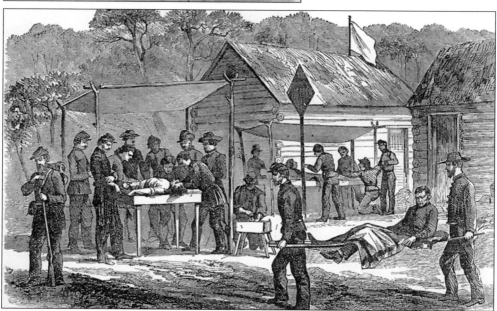

This depiction of an aid station illustrates the plan Dr. Blair described during the Battle of Stone's River or Murfreesboro. At the far table, there are three or four assistants and a surgeon. The nearer table may be a consultation about an amputation. The mini-balls used during the Civil War caused severe bone damage, making amputations unavoidable when blood vessels were severely damaged. (HW)

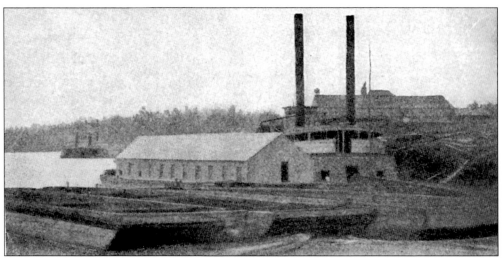

Some victims of smallpox were quarantined on barges such as this one on the Mississippi. Dr. William Gillespie of the 83rd Indiana Infantry was assigned to smallpox patients. While most regiments were vaccinated for small pox, the disease was responsible for 4,717 deaths in Union hospitals. Although the germ theory was not understood at the time of the Civil War, the practice of quarantining those with smallpox was employed. (MPH)

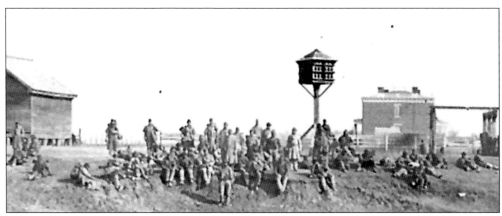

These convalescent African-American soldiers are recovering at Aiken's Landing, Virginia. The Aiken's house is on the right. African-American troops experienced higher rates of respiratory diseases and continued fevers than did white troops. On average, an African-American soldier was sick 3.3 times per year and a white soldier 2.4. (Courtesy of the Library of Congress)

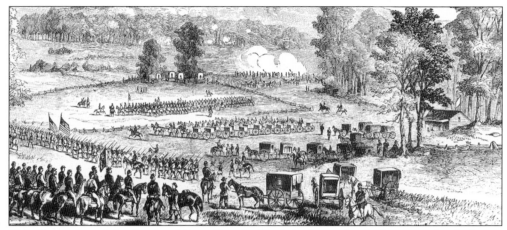

This illustration of the Battle of Cross Keys in Virginia shows the deployment of ambulances before a battle. Misappropriation of ambulances for the carrying of personnel baggage and even the surgeons themselves was a common charge leveled against surgeons. Infirm soldiers and those convalescing were allowed to ride in ambulances rather than marching. Assignment as ambulance driver often meant that the driver could at least sleep under the wagon when no other shelter was available. (HW)

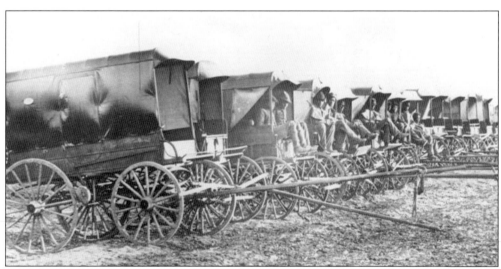

An Indiana firm, Damron and March, manufactured 50 ambulances for the army. Ambulances were uncomfortable at best. On the rocky, hilly roads of Tennessee and Kentucky, they were tortuous. The first army models had two wheels, while later ambulances were designed with four wheels. Stretchers were suspended from rubber straps inside hospital trains that acted as shock absorbers. Ambulances were considered superior to army wagons by the wounded. (MPH)

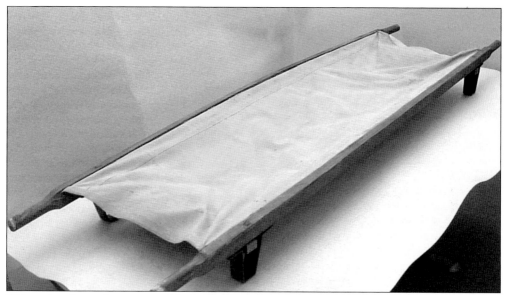

This style of stretcher was used by both Confederate and Union forces during the Civil War. After and during battles musicians and chaplains were assigned to bring the wounded off the field. When a soldier was wounded in battle his comrades, who were often his friends, neighbors, or relatives, rushed to assist him off the field. This left the regiment two or three men short instead of one. Men were ordered to leave the wounded where they lay. (Courtesy of the National Museum of Civil War Medicine)

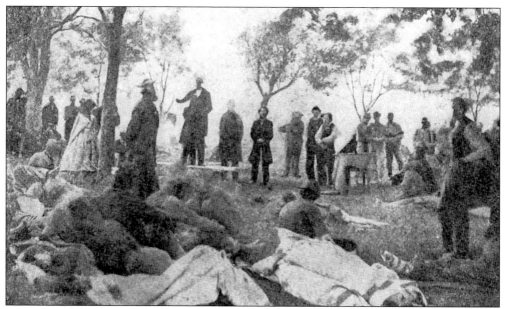

This scene shows the medical staff pausing during their care of the wounded at Spotsylvania for a prayer or blessing from a chaplain. Suffering was felt to be necessary to a perfected spiritual life, and the patience with which the afflicted bore their suffering was believed to be pivotal to their spiritual salvation. Even young children were expected to suffer without complaint. There was extreme pressure on soldiers to endure their suffering bravely. (MPH)

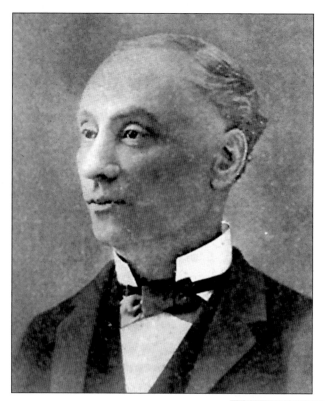

Robert N. Todd was born in Lexington, Kentucky. He served in Missouri with the 26th Indiana Infantry as surgeon. His words at a meeting of the Indiana State Medical Society show us that not all Civil War surgeons believed in the miraculous powers of the drug calomel. When asked to comment on 10 grain doses of calomel, he stated: "There can be no doubt that patients do sometimes get well after being subjected to such enormous doses of calomel. God is good." (K)

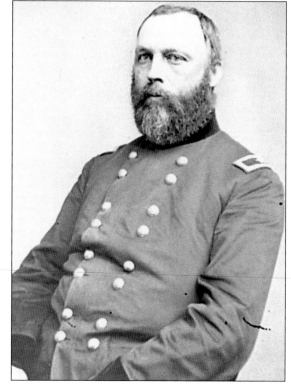

Brigadier General William A. Hammond was Surgeon General of the U.S. Army during the Civil War. He issued a very controversial order that limited the use of calomel, mercurous chloride, by surgeons. Calomel was erroneously believed to alleviate diarrhea and other stomach complaints. Too much calomel caused the teeth to fall out, the gums to rot, and even caused damage to the jaw bone. Hammond was courtmartialed but exonerated after the war. (Courtesy of the Library of Congress)

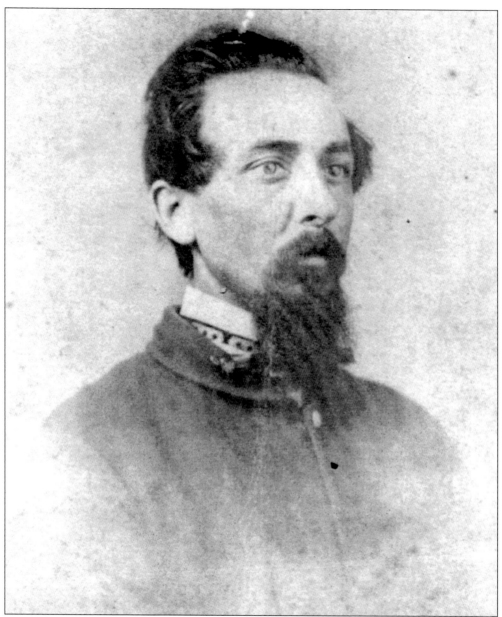

Edmond L. Castator of the 9th Indiana Cavalry was mustered in as hospital steward with no apparent medical background. After the war, he was employed by and lived with his brother-in-law in Brooklyn, New York. Castator's employer and relative claimed he was a man of intemperate habits who fired a gun in his house, didn't want to work, and tried to set fire to his home. Castator's habits did not shorten his life; he died in a Soldier's Home at 97. While it is unknown whether he was abusing alcohol during the war, one Hoosier soldier was known to ask, "How would you like to take medicine issued by a steward so drunk that his tongue was very thick and he could hardly stand?" (Courtesy of John Sickles)

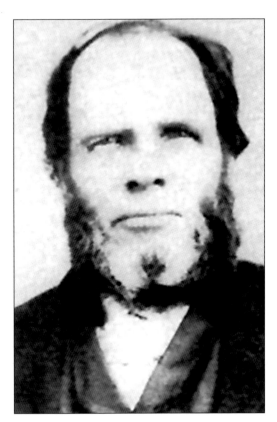

David Hutchinson of Putnam County was born in Lesmehaga, Scotland. He started his study of medicine in Glasgow and came to America in 1829. He continued to study medicine at Medical College of Ohio in Cincinnati, and eventually became president of the state medical association. Although he was the surgeon of the 30th for only a few months, he left an account of the medical situation in Murfreesboro after the Battle of Stone's River. (RLML)

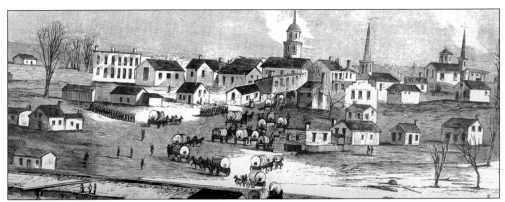

At Murfreesboro, Hutchinson reported that serious cases were left there at division hospital while other cases were moved to hospitals in Nashville, Tennessee. Flap amputations were left open to heal without dressings. Nearly all the secondary amputations died. He also reported that measles were disastrous if not immediately treated with brandy and quinine. (HW)

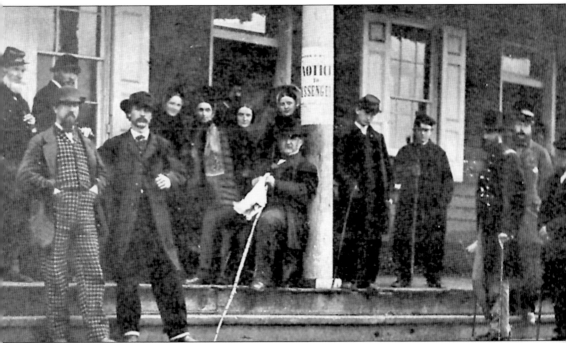

Railroads were very important during the Civil War. This group at a train stations in Hanover, Virginia, must resemble groups of Hoosiers gathered to visit their ill or wounded relatives. Finding soldiers who were not with their regiments was not always easy. Dr. Hutchinson was a military agent in Nashville. His office kept track of Indiana soldiers in the hospitals there and assisted families who were looking for their loved ones. In February 1863, he informed the citizens of Indiana that they could not pass south of Nashville except by way of Memphis. However, he stated Indiana citizens still came to Nashville seeking sons and husbands only 30 miles away but across a line over which civilians were not allowed to pass. Room and board was $2–3 dollars per day and no one's influence could get them to see their relatives. He also warned fathers not to take their sons from hospitals unless they had been officially discharged. Only the surgeon in charge could issue a discharge. (MPH)

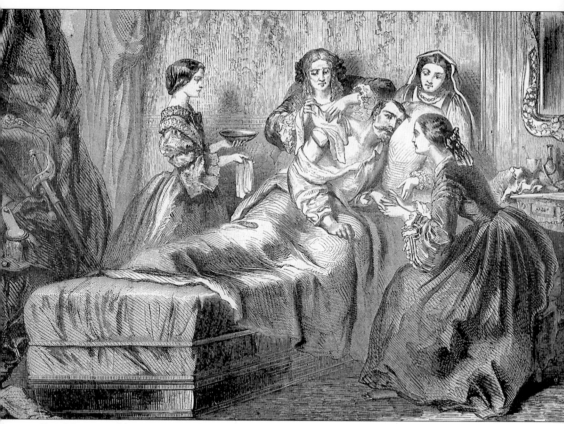

Few Hoosier soldiers imagined being wounded or ill when they marched away from home. If they thought of being a wounded hero, they saw themselves surrounded by loving female relatives attending to their every need. Women were the caregivers in Victorian society. Male nurses, no matter how dedicated, were held suspect by patients. Gender roles may have also influenced the relationship of the caregiver surgeons and the traditional male roles of the other regimental officers. Governor Morton sent parties of female nurses to many other hospitals. They often performed the duties of cooks and laundry attendants. Women serving with the Christian Commission also helped the hospitalized, and several orders of Catholic sisters volunteered for duty at various hospitals. A female presence was considered conducive to healing. (RLML)

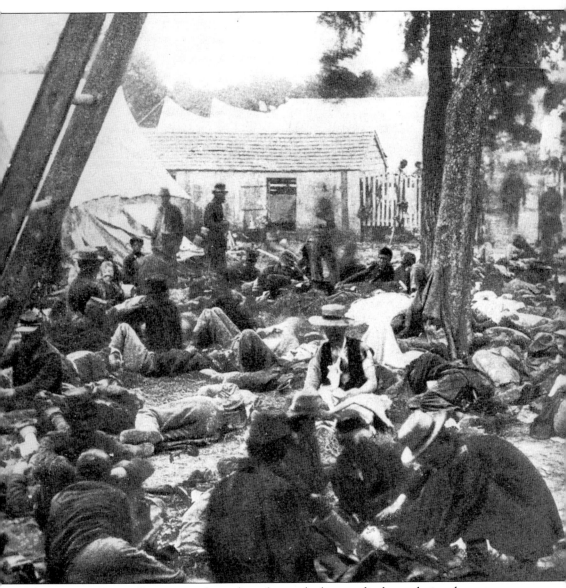

This scene at Savage Station was the reality of even the best medical care during the war—too many wounded and too few caregivers. Hospitals, no matter how well run and orderly, were not like home. Caring for one family member was far different from caring for 100 patients in a makeshift ward. People at the scene of battles or at large hospitals reminded those sending supplies that a bushel of apples might do for treats for a family for weeks but did little for a hospital of 100 men. Opiates were available to treat pain. The opium derivative, laudanum, was often used as a home remedy either alone or in compounds. The anesthetic chloroform was used during operations. However, without devices to monitor a patient's vital signs, physicians were extremely careful not to administer a lethal dose. Whiskey was given to make bitter quinine more palatable and as a restorative. (MPH)

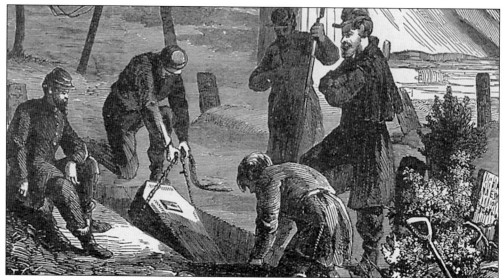

Burial at home "among friends" was expected for fallen war heroes. Towns often sent committees to return the bodies to their hometowns for burial. Advertisers suggested that metallic coffins were useful for this purpose. Bodies were often hastily buried and not disinterred until months later, making identification difficult. In the Eastern Theater of the war, bodies were buried with personal identification in bottles so that remains could later be correctly identified. (HW)

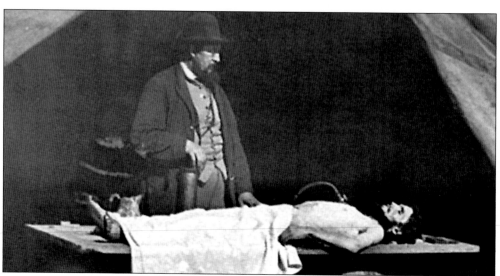

Embalming was not an option for most families when they lost a loved one in the war, reality dictating that remains be buried hastily near where they died without the embalming expense. Returning remains to distant states was also not practical. There are many eyewitness accounts of remains staying unburied years after the Battle of the Wilderness. Dr. Lewis Humphreys personally embalmed one of St. Joseph's County's soldiers early in the war. (MPH)

Four

WOMEN'S WORK

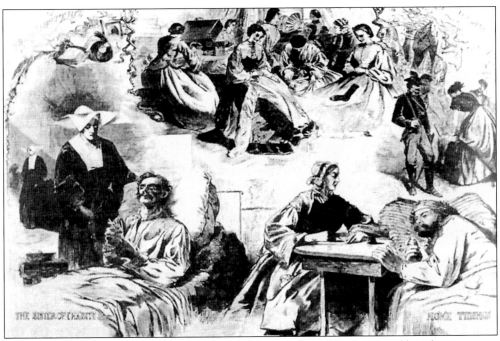

The many roles women played to support the soldiers in the field are pictured here by a post-war artist. Thousands of unnamed Hoosier women toiled, economized, and retrenched to supply food and clothing to soldiers and patients in hospitals throughout the country. They turned their own clothes into shirts, underclothing, and bandages. Women stripped their homes of bedding to supply hospitals. Mary Livermore, head of the Chicago Sanitary Commission, requested one box of hospital supplies per month from each ladies aid committee. Some women who contributed to these supply efforts also tended the farms their husbands left in their care while at war. Washerwoman and cook were two roles which allowed women to travel with the army. (HW)

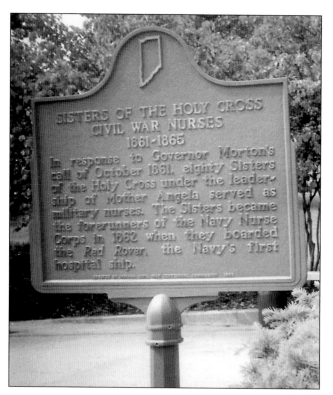

This historic marker honors the Sisters of the Holy Cross of South Bend, some of the first Civil War nurses. The sisters were the first nurses on the *Red Rover*. The sisters were preferred to "Protestant" women by military doctors. They were obedient and unquestioning. Women such as Mary Livermore, Mary Bickerdyke, and Eliza George were used to ruling their homes and were not so submissive. (Courtesy of Geneva McKenzie)

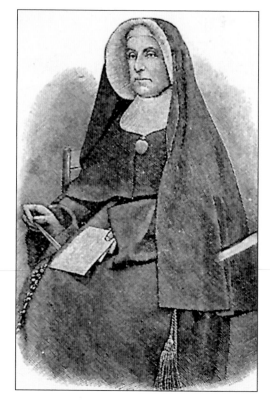

Mother Mary of St. Angela of the Sisters of the Holy Cross, Notre Dame, Indiana, sent six sisters to Cairo, Illinois, and then six more to Paducah, Kentucky. In Cairo, the sisters met future General Grant. Mother Mary Angela was a cousin of General Sherman by marriage. Another contingent from this convent was sent to Mound City, Illinois. They also nursed at a pest hospital in Missouri and the Naval Hospital in Memphis. (OAN)

Mrs. Mary Watson of Indianapolis went to Nashville Hospital No. 14 after the Battle of Stone's River. She witnessed the deaths of 30 patients per day in the weeks after the battle. After catching typhoid fever herself, she went home. She went to a field hospital in Murfreesboro where, as the only white woman, she noted that African-American women there did the cooking and washing. In Murfreesboro, she found her own husband critically ill. (OAN)

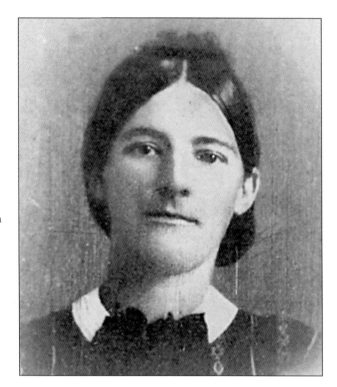

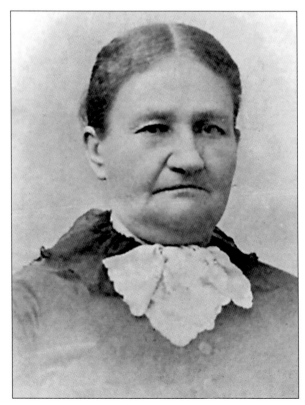

Mary Baker of Concord, Indiana, was a cook in the special diet kitchen of Officers' Hospital No. 2 in Nashville. During the Battle of Nashville, shells shook the building. She says, "I met two soldier girls in blue. One, Frances Hook, alias Harry Miller, who served two years and nine months; the other was called Anna. She was put under my charge until the military authorities could send her North." (OAN)

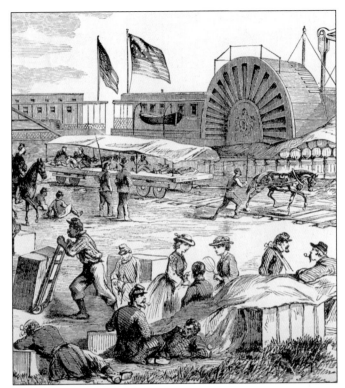

Scenes similar to this at Fortress Monroe occurred on the wharves of Madison, New Albany, Jeffersonville, and Evansville, as side-wheeler steamers unloaded cargoes of sick and wounded soldiers. Women waited on the docks and at train stations throughout Indiana to offer tea, coffee, and water to the suffering passengers. Telegrams were sent to cities and towns where the wounded were expected to arrive. (HW)

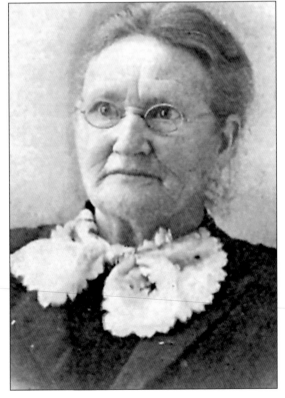

Elizabeth Hunt was living in Iowa, where she took charge of the care of patients at a smallpox hospital. She was stricken with smallpox herself. The government denied her pension because she had not served for six months. She later lived in Bloomingdale, Indiana. Since nurses were not usually sworn into service, many women who gave their lives and health in service to their country were denied pensions that many undeserving men received. (OAN)

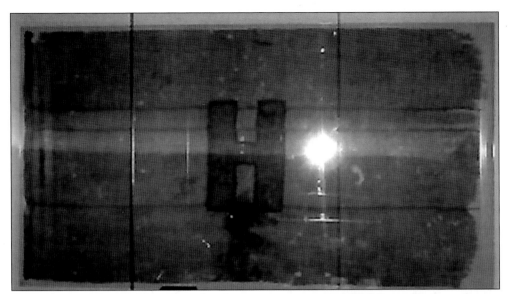

Hospitals were identified by yellow flags bearing a green capital "H." Several Indiana doctors wrote from Paducah, Kentucky, to the women of New Albany in 1861: "We are in want of a good hospital flag, which will indicate the spot where the sick and wounded federal soldiers are cared for. The flag should be about 6 by 9 feet, yellow color, and of good material." (Courtesy of the National Museum of Civil War Medicine)

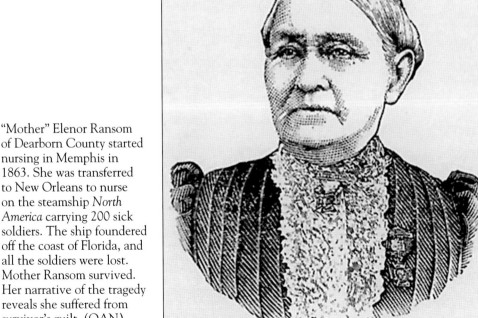

"Mother" Elenor Ransom of Dearborn County started nursing in Memphis in 1863. She was transferred to New Orleans to nurse on the steamship *North America* carrying 200 sick soldiers. The ship foundered off the coast of Florida, and all the soldiers were lost. Mother Ransom survived. Her narrative of the tragedy reveals she suffered from survivor's guilt. (OAN)

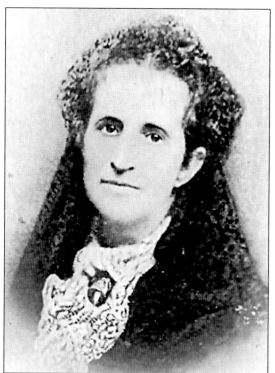

Dr. Mary Ellis with her husband raised a company of the 1st Missouri. She accompanied her husband, the colonel, in her own carriage with two African-American servants to assist her nursing. At the Battle of Pea Ridge, she stood by the operating table for hours until she fainted. Unfortunately, her only son was maimed in the war and preceded her in death. She earned a medical degree in 1857, and practiced in Indianapolis for many years. (OAN)

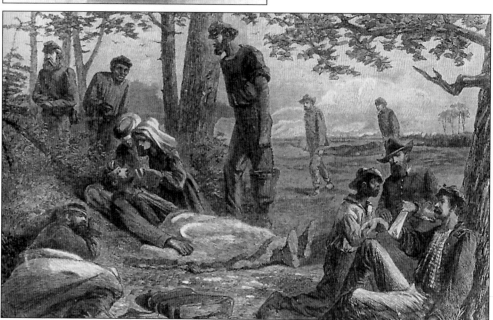

The Goshen Democrat in 1862 carried the following quote: "It is a noble sight, [to see] a highly educated lady accustomed to every indulgence that wealth can furnish, thus employed with disordered hair; hoopless, in a soiled calico dress bespattered with blood, coal-smut, and grease, forgetting every feeling but the one of seeking and helping the most wretched and neglected: God has blessed my eyes with the sight of such a one. The name of the noble-minded lady shall not soon be forgotten." (HW)

Dr. Mary Walker, pictured here, was controversial for her attire that included trousers. Dr. Mary Frame Thomas and Dr. Cloe Annette Buckel of Indiana served in near obscurity during the war. Dr. Thomas took supplies to Vicksburg and nursed 50 wounded and sick soldiers on the return trip. Dr. Buckel supervised nurses in Memphis, Tennessee, and the large hospital in Jeffersonville. After the war, she went to California where she founded San Francisco Women's Hospital. (Courtesy of the Library of Congress)

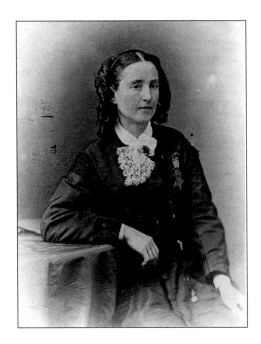

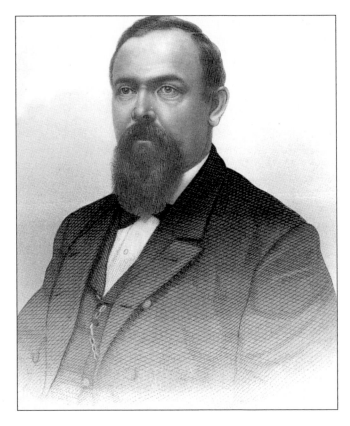

Oliver P. Morton, governor, started the Indiana Sanitary Commission, not trusting the U.S. Sanitary Commission to appropriately or efficiently distribute supplies and aid to Indiana troops. Hoosiers were active in the U.S. Sanitary Commission, the Cincinnati Sanitary Commission, the Northwest Sanitary Commission, and the St. Louis Sanitary Commission. Morton commissioned his own nurses who often had to defend their places in hospitals where the nurses were commissioned by Dorothea Dix. (RLML)

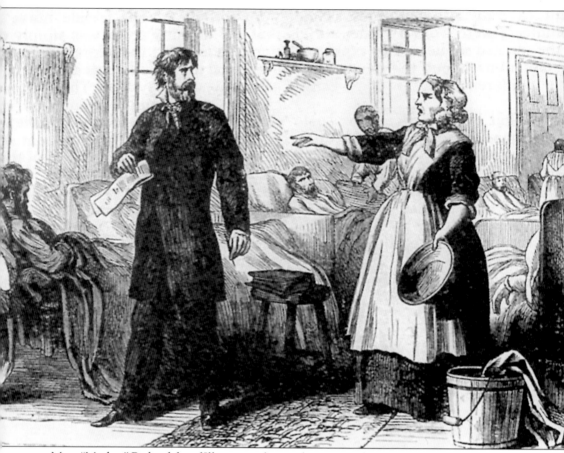

Mary "Mother" Bickerdyke of Illinois was known by many Indiana soldiers. From Ft. Donelson to Lookout Mountain, she was undaunted by conflicts with surgeons, army officers, and impossible conditions. She even defied General Sherman's ban on women traveling with the army on his march through Georgia. This scene depicts a confrontation between Bickerdyke and a surgeon she considers irresponsible or careless. She and her assistants made gallons of coffee. Her many years of service during the war were not immediately recognized with a pension. Bickerdyke's calico dress and sunbonnet were sold for $100 as war souvenirs soon after the war. (HW)

Mary Venard of Wabash was commissioned a nurse through the Indiana Sanitary Commission. At the Howard School Hospital in Nashville, Tennessee, she was in charge of the diet kitchen and nursing. She then served at the Marine Hospital in Natchez. After Natchez, Venard returned home and was soon called to Indianapolis to work in the refugee home and the ladies home. The Morton G.A.R. Post presented her with the pin she wears. (OAN)

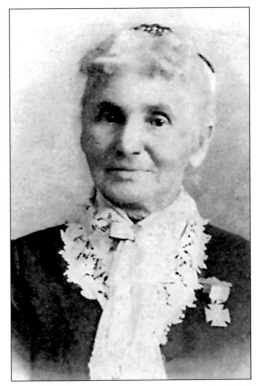

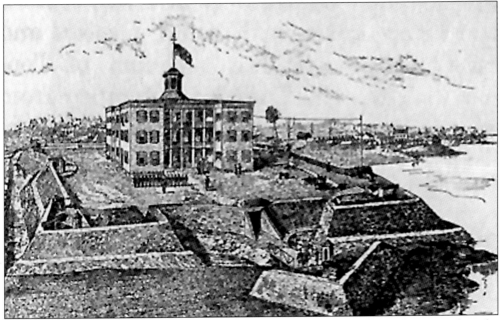

At Hospital No. 1 in Paducah, Kentucky, Almira Fifield of Valparaiso, Indiana, "sank under labors for the sick and wounded soldiers. Her death was the result of congestive chills . . . Having had a thorough medical education, she devoted her talents and acquirements so faithfully and modestly to the soldiers' benefit, that only her skill discovered her profession, as she held the position alone, of female nurse, under the Chicago Sanitary Commission." (HW)

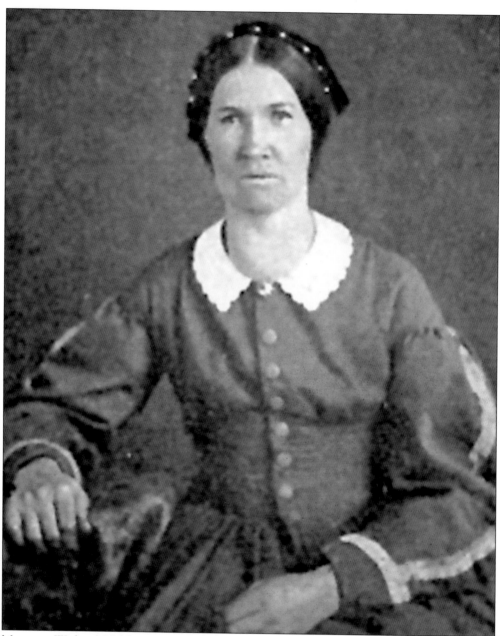

Margaret Wishard Noble was a sister of Joseph and William Henry Wishard. Her mother organized her Presbyterian women's church sewing circle into a soldiers' aid society. Women's missionary groups in churches often became aid societies during the Civil War. Such aid groups sent hospital supplies to regiments. They also raised money for soldier's families who became destitute. Some groups in Indiana were run entirely by women and others had men in the positions of leadership. One knitting circle told the men who wished to attend that their hands would be employed in winding yarn for the knitters. All who attended were charged 5¢ or 10¢, and the money went towards the purchase of more yarn for knitting socks. Socks, especially early in the war, were not supplied by the military and it was the knitting needles of the women that kept the army moving. (RLML)

Lois Dennett Dunbar attended the wounded from Fort Donelson with Mrs. Harriet Colfax of Michigan City. She offered aid as the wounded were taken from the boats. Later, she was sent to Hospital No. 2 in Evansville and gained charge of four other hospitals there. Unlike many Indiana nurses, she was commissioned by Dorothea Dix. She describes passing out treats to patients and also assisting in amputations. She married a patient who she claims was saved by her nursing. (OAN)

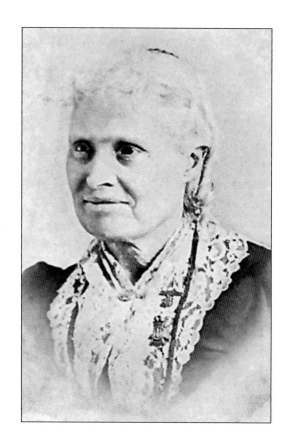

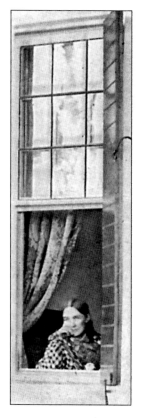

Women left at home could spend hours sewing shirts, canning fruits, and writing letters. There were still many hours to ponder their life should the men not return from war. Communities recognized that many soldiers' families were in dire need of assistance while their men were away at war; often those families faced starvation, homelessness, and degradation. In Indiana, many towns formed committees to look after the welfare of these families in peril. (MPH)

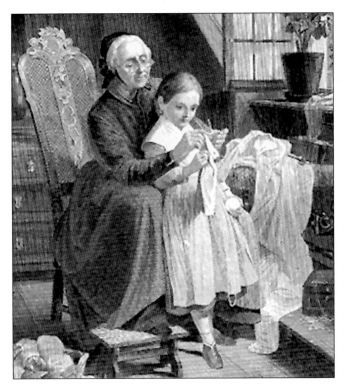

The men marched off to war, and Indiana women picked up their knitting needles. The army was unable to supply the socks for soldiers. Women sent their handiwork to someone they knew in the army or to a company raised in their own community, to a local aid group, or to the Indiana Sanitary Commission. Although some soldiers reported the loss of sanitary supplies through theft, most encouraged women to keep sending needed extras. (Copyright Hope Greenberg, University of Vermont. Used by permission)

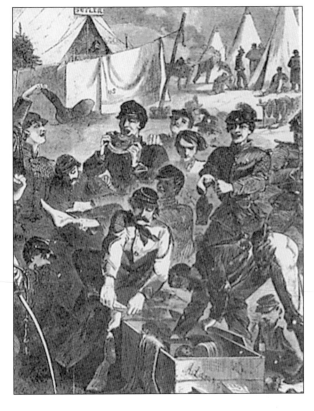

In this scene, soldiers joyfully examine and consume the contents of a box from home. The soldier on the right seems to have worn out the seat of his trousers. Another rejoices in socks. More than treats, these boxes from home supplied many items that were either very expensive at the sutler's tent or unavailable. Socks, mittens, gloves, and scarves were especially needed in the winter. (HW)

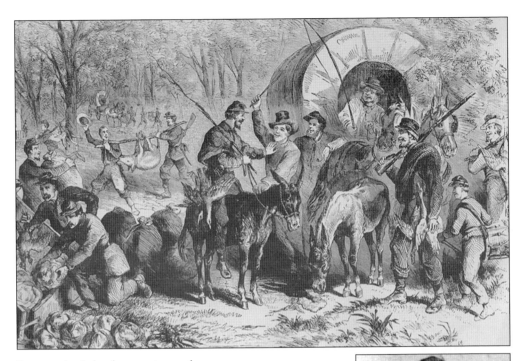

Foraging by federal troops in southern states was necessary to the health of the troops. A diet of hardtack, salt pork, and coffee would lead to scurvy, now known to be caused by a vitamin C deficiency. Fresh fruit and vegetables as well as fresh meat contained vitamins necessary to the health of soldiers in the field. Civil War diaries contain many stories of finding blackberries on the march, which are good for preventing gastric disorders. Edwin W. High of the 68th Indiana said blackberries were used as food and medicine. However, the soldiers' diet was not the surgeons' responsibility. Packages from home and aid societies containing sauerkraut and pickles were another way to supply essential vitamins. Of course, the troops didn't realize this when they craved pickles and kraut. (HW)

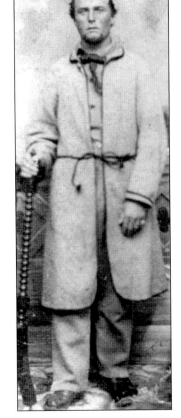

Private Edward Lonie of the 2nd Illinois had his photo taken in a hospital coat. Items such as these coats were made by women for aid societies. One Indianapolis doctor to be, Joseph Eastman, attended medical classes at Georgetown University while at a hospital at Washington D.C. (Photograph by Wallis G. Lonie Jr. Collection at USAMHI)

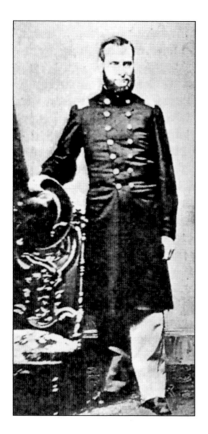

Pictured is Colonel Abel Streight of the 51st Indiana Infantry. On December 20, 1861, in Bardstown, Kentucky, Colonel Streight's wife faced the task of assisting Dr. E. Collins in caring for 125 men suffering with measles. Hospital supplies were not included in the regiment's supplies at this point in the war. Officers' wives often accompanied troops into the field and acted as unofficial nurses. (RLML)

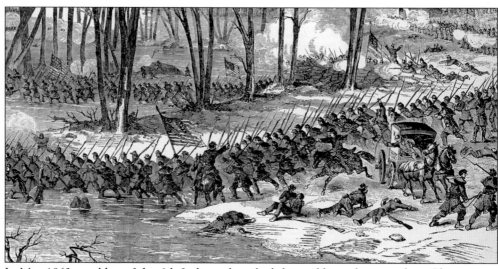

In May 1863, a soldier of the 6th Indiana described the wedding of a nurse from Chicago to a private from the 15th Indiana. The wedding party toured part of the Murfreesboro battlefield at Stone's River in the company of several high ranking Union officers. Several female nurses married their patients or hospital stewards. Pictured is the Murfreesboro battlefield. On the right is an ambulance. (HW)

Five

WAR STORIES

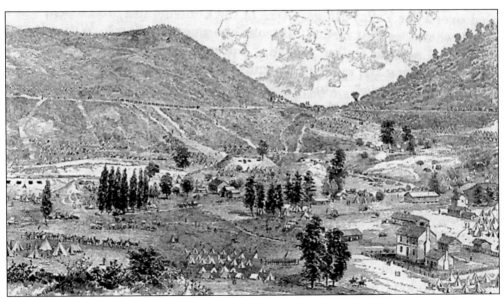

The 49th Indiana experienced sickness in the isolated area around the Cumberland Gap in Kentucky. Colonel Ray wrote to Governor Morton of his regiment's situation, and received the following reply from Governor Morton: "Colonel Ray—The Governor will send you a lot of supplies and two additional surgeons, immediately via Lexington. Never hesitate to call on us for any assistance. It will be promptly given. W.R. Holloway, Private Secretary to Governor Morton." (HW)

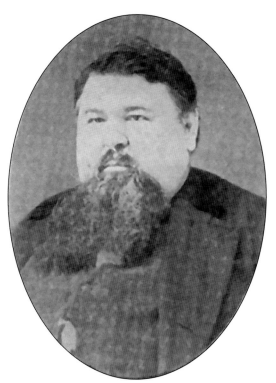

Four surgeons and four assistant surgeons of the 49th Indiana Infantry resigned before Emmanuel Hawn received his commission as surgeon. The 49th had at one time over 400 sick men and no commissioned medical officer. Several line officers with medical experience cared for the ill while doing their duties as captains and lieutenants. William Z. Smith rose from private to hospital steward, to assistant surgeon, to surgeon before resigning. Hawn succeeded him. (RLML)

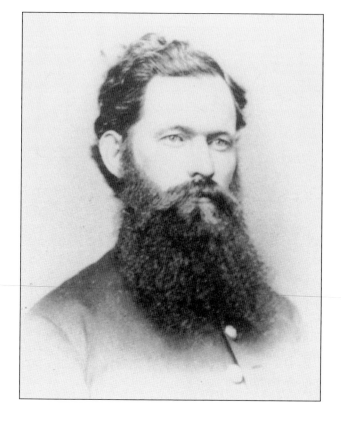

Edward Buzette of Switzerland County was assistant surgeon and surgeon of the 49th. Several men appointed medical officers became ill themselves. Frantic letters written by the 49th's colonel and colonel's wife to Governor Morton requested the appointment of specific individuals to the medical staff. They finally wrote, "We want a good competent Surgeon and are in considerable need of such." (Courtesy of the Indiana State Library, Manuscripts Section, Picture Collection)

Assistant Surgeon Asa McKinney of the 31st Indiana Infantry was taken prisoner at the Battle of Murfreesboro. Surgeons of both sides frequently fell into the enemy hands. The sick and wounded could not be moved so surgeons and medical staff had to stay behind. Surgeons were considered non-combatants. Enlisted men such as hospital stewards could be sent to such prisons as Andersonville. McKinney lived in Washington County. (Courtesy of USAMHI)

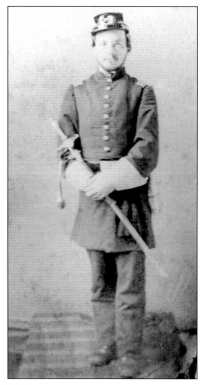

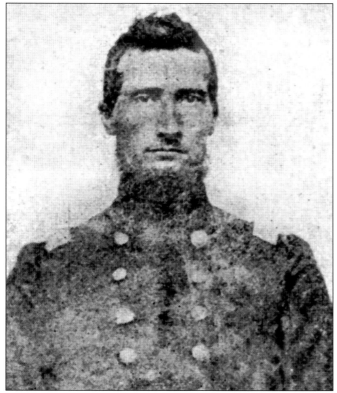

Jarvis J. Johnson of the 27th Indiana was with Federal troops when they entered Winchester, Virginia. There the remains of one of John Brown's sons, Watson, were found on display at the medical school. Johnson shipped the exhibit to Martinsville, Indiana, and displayed it in his office for 20 years. The story varies, as one states he had it in the garret. In 1880, the remains were buried by the Brown family in New York. (Regimental History)

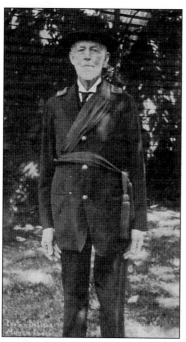

Dr. General William Harrison Kemper addressed young Indiana doctors about to leave for World War I. He reminded them that the doctors of the 1860's were brave and dedicated. They had lacked the support of trained nurses, the Red Cross, and of an organized Army Medical Department. He also pointed out that at the time of the Civil War there was no medical school in Indiana. (RLML)

Found in central Tennessee, this artifact puzzled the finders as to its inscription and original use. Expert advice confirmed that it is the handle from the dress sword of a hospital steward. "Tip" was General William Harrison Kemper's nickname, based on the presidential campaign slogan of General William Harrison, "Tippecanoe and Tyler, Too." How the sword handle came to be discarded is not known. (RLML)

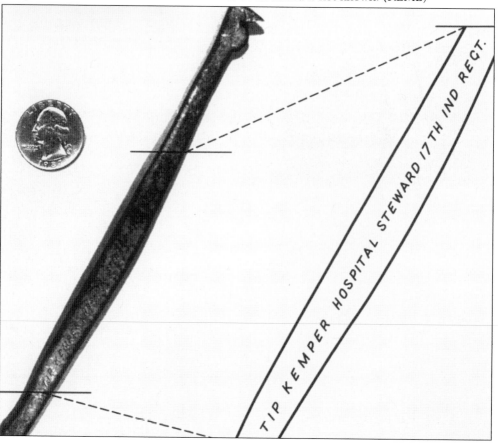

(*Right*) Mrs. G.W.H. Kemper was married to the doctor soon after the war. Kemper may have carried this picture during the Civil War. She shared his life in Muncie, Indiana, for many decades. Many widows of Civil War surgeons received pensions well into the 20th century. As early as 1862 ads appeared in local papers for agents who would assist the families of deceased soldiers in their quest for pensions. (RLML)

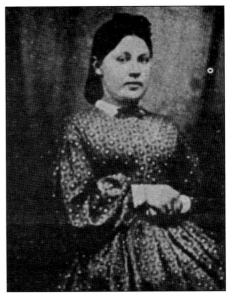

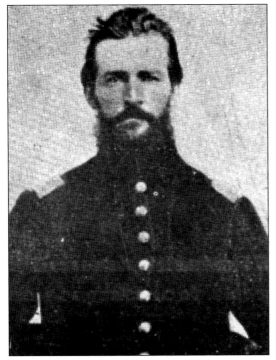

(*Left*) G.W.H. Kemper was a private in the 7th Indiana Infantry for six months. He joined the 17th Indiana Infantry as hospital steward and was promoted to assistant surgeon with no medical experience. Leaving his unit before the end of the war, he attended Long Island Medical School. (RLML)

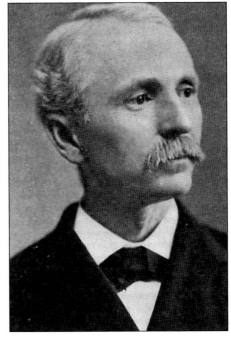

Samuel E. Munford was a private, then hospital steward, then assistant surgeon, and finally surgeon of the 17th Indiana Infantry. He later became brigade surgeon of Wilder's Brigade. He was a pupil of W.W. Blair and graduated from Jefferson Medical College in 1861. Dr. Kemper was associated with Samuel Munford for three years, and said that he loved him "as Jonathan loved David." (K)

81

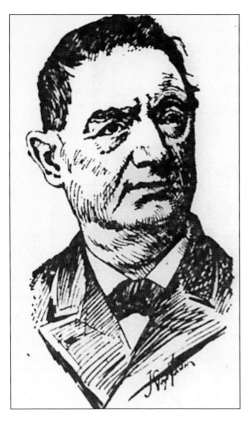

Alexander Mullen was surgeon of the 35th Indiana, the Irish regiment. He began his medical studies while a cabin boy. The assistant surgeon of the 35th was Dr. Averdick of Landau, Rhenish Bavaria. Alexander's wife was daughter of Baron H. Carl Hudler of Kaiserheim, Landau, Rhenish Bavaria. The baron received the cross of the Legion of Honor from Napoleon, for his services as a surgeon during the Russian campaign. (Courtesy of the Indiana State Library, Manuscripts Section, Picture Collection)

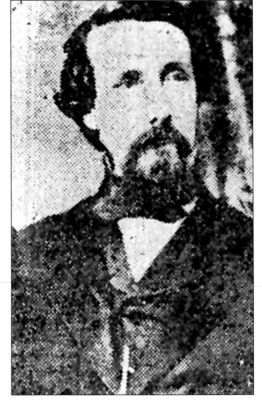

Alexander's brother, Bernard Mullen, also trained as a physician and eventually was appointed colonel of the 35th Irish Regiment. As a youth, Colonel Mullen went off to the Mexican War when the citizens of Versailles, Indiana, caught him in the process of body snatching for the benefit of his medical studies. A third Mullen brother was also a physician, serving in the War of Texas Independence. Colonel Alexander Mullen eventually died of tuberculosis. (Courtesy of the Indiana State Library, Manuscripts Section, Picture Collection)

The son of surgeon Alexander Mullen, Bernard, was adjutant of the 35th. He was killed at Dobbyn's Ford, Tennessee. Soon after the death of his son, Surgeon Mullen tried to be transferred to the hospital in Madison, Indiana. Another son, Alexander Junior, became a doctor, following in his father's footsteps. (Courtesy of the Indiana State Library, Manuscripts Section, Picture Collection)

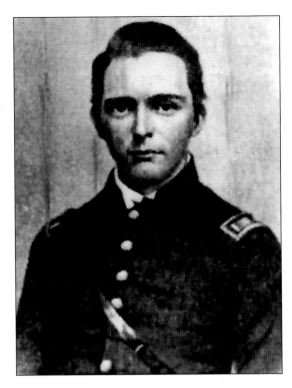

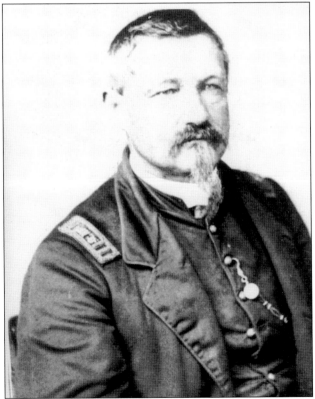

Emil Forstmeyer was an assistant surgeon in the 32nd Indiana Infantry or the First German Regiment. Forstmeyer was born in Germany and educated in Berlin. He practiced in Blairsville and Mount Vernon. Those citizens supported him when he wrote to Governor Morton, in German, for a commission. Indiana fielded only two ethnic regiments—the Irish and German. (Courtesy of the Indiana State Library, Manuscripts Section, Picture Collection)

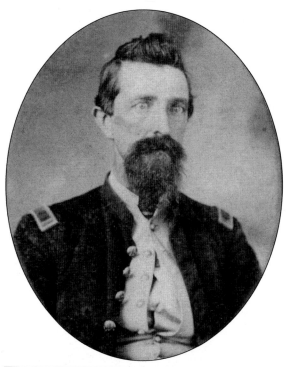

Jacob Montieth of Lynn, Indiana, was second assistant surgeon of the 69th. He treated a little girl in Mobile, Alabama, who was the daughter of the local newspaper owner. She recovered from the fever that had caused her parents great concern. Ironically, Dr. Monteith died at his home October 29, 1865, of "entrentic" fever. (Courtesy of civilwarindiana.com)

CONSOLIDATED MORNING REPORT of																														**Regiment of**			

This interesting note appears on a copy of a morning report of the 69th regiment: "Surgeon—Slow but industrious (referring to David Evans); 1st Assistant Surgeon—Absent since fight at Vicksburg—no reason known (Witt); 2nd Assistant Surgeon—Present—best of the lot (Monteith); Chaplain Worth 4 doctors. Hospital—No Right accommodations—Sick at General Hospital; Pretty good supply of medicine; Camp—Tolerably dry." (Courtesy of the Indiana State Archives, Commission on Public Records)

A section of a pontoon bridge such as this was being used as a ferry at Bayou McHenry near Indianola, Texas. When the middle pontoon sank, the occupants of the raft were thrown with full equipment into wind-churned water. Surgeon Witt and 10 others of the 69th Indiana, along with up to 20 African-American ferrymen, drowned. One member of the 1st Indiana Heavy Artillery found a plank and swam to the middle of the bay, making several rescue trips. (MPH)

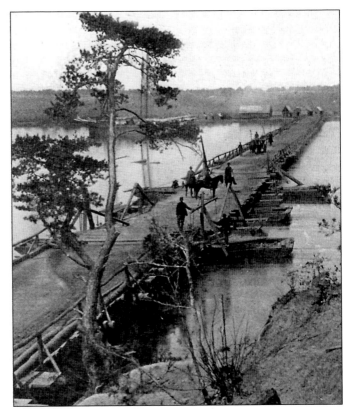

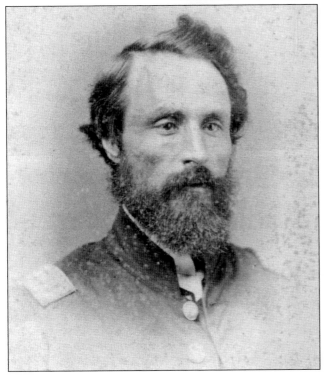

Dr. William B. Witt of Dublin, Indiana, assistant surgeon of the 69th Indiana, was no stranger to danger. In 1857, he had gone as a missionary for the Methodist Church in West Africa. He left his African mission due to fever contracted there, and drowned as the regiment was crossing a bayou on the coast of Texas. Witt's last words were reported to have been in prayer and praise of God. (Courtesy of civilwarindiana.com)

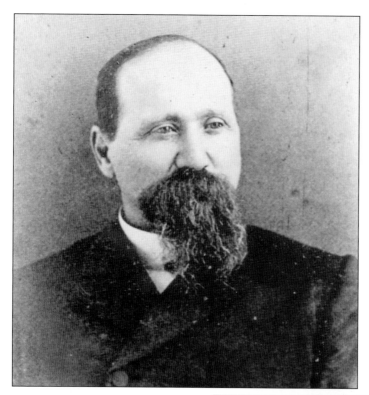

David Swarts, first assistant surgeon of the 100th, was originally a captain. He graduated from Ohio Medical College in 1860, and in 1862 married Vesta Swarts. The regimental history reports he was several times detached to corps hospitals after heavy engagements. He enjoyed the distinction of being one of the best surgeons of the 15 th Corps, although the regimental correspondence indicates he was absent without leave and "did not behave well." (Regimental History)

Dr. Swarts' bride, Vesta, went to Louisville and found a post in one of the hospitals there to be closer to her husband. After working at two Louisville hospitals, she was discharged due to ill health. After the war, she attended medical school and practiced for 23 years in Auburn, Indiana. Although they did not serve together, this couple gave several years of their lives to military service. (OAN)

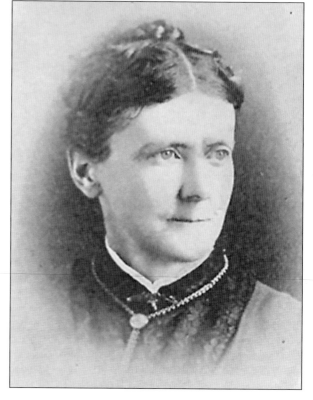

Henry H. Hand was a private before being promoted to hospital steward of the 100th. He was ambushed at Peay's Ferry road in the Carolinas and then taken to prison in Florence, South Carolina. Richard Magee or McGee was recommended highly from his work in the camps in Indianapolis and commissioned the 100th's second assistant surgeon. Later Magee was dismissed because he had been a prisoner in the Illinois State prison. (Regimental History)

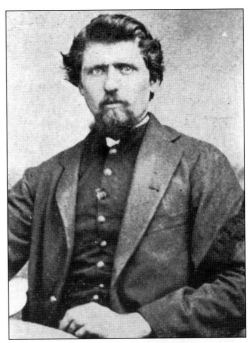

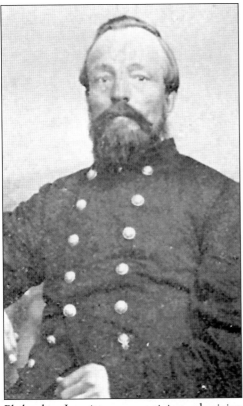

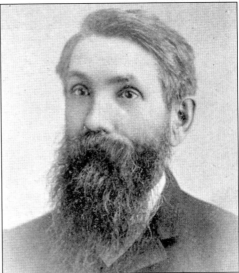

Philander Leavitt, a practicing physician before the war, enlisted as a private in the 100th Indiana Infantry. He worked his way up to surgeon of the regiment with the support of the officers and men. His son was originally a member of the 100th, but transferred to the 48th regiment. The 100th lost 56 enlisted men to mortal wounds and 173 to disease. (Regimental History)

Dr. Samuel France, surgeon of the 100th, wrote, "I find, as I expected, that the position of hospital surgeon is no sinecure. I, and those associated with me in the medical department of the 100th, are doing all in our power to alleviate the sufferings of those under our charge, and we are left little leisure for social correspondence." His comrades said he spread cheery works and jokes that often did more good than his pills. He practiced for many years in Bourbon, Indiana. (Regimental History)

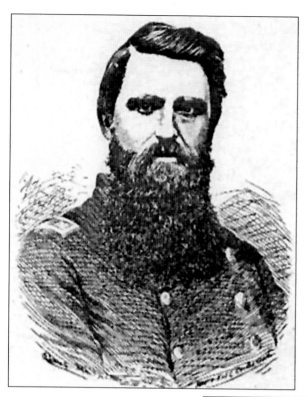

Dr. John H. Rerick was the author of his regimental history. He was with the 44th Indiana at Shiloh, Corinth, Boonville, Iuka, and Stones River, Chickamauga, and Chattanooga to the end of the war. He was editor and proprietor of the Lagrange *Standard* newspaper. The 44th Indiana Infantry lost 76 men to mortal wounds and 220 to disease. (Regimental History)

James K. Bigelow of Grant County and Indianapolis was the assistant surgeon to the 8th Indiana Infantry. He married, went back to the war, became a widower, married his dead wife's sister, returned to war, and became a widower again. The 8th was stationed in West Virginia, Arkansas, Mississippi, and Texas. Bigelow published a history of the 8th in 1864. Other published accounts praise his attention to the men under his care. At the close of the war, he married a widow. (Courtesy of civilwarindiana.com)

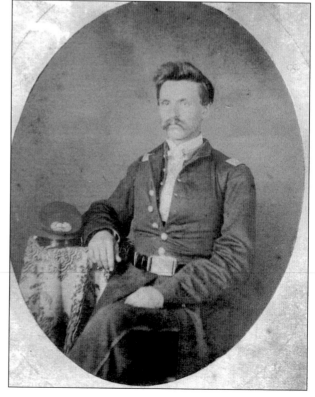

Dr. William Henry Wishard (see pages 10 and 20) was a volunteer surgeon sent by Governor Morton to supplement the regimental medical staff. After the surrender of Vicksburg he was greeted by a Confederate soldier, who told him that every morning for a week he had shot at him as he walked from his tent to the field hospital in a white coat. The doctor's calm response was, "That would explain why I heard so many bullets whizzing past my ears." (RLML)

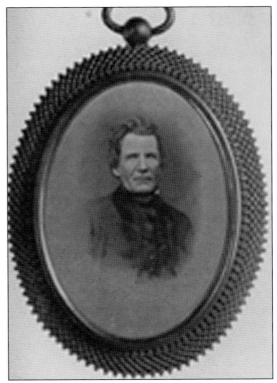

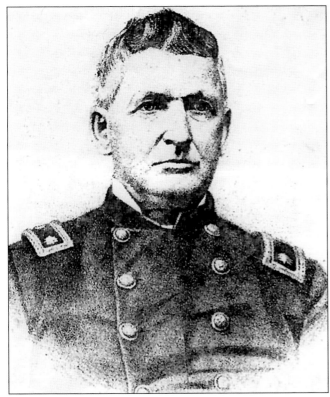

James L. Morrow, 72nd Indiana Infantry, told that 1,300 wounded were admitted to his hospital after a battle near Crab Orchard, Kentucky. After spending three months in charge of the Frankfort, Kentucky, hospitals, he acted as brigade surgeon during Wheeler's Raid. This raid furnished rapid skirmishes, and finally culminated in the severe and decisive engagement at Farmington. On account of ill health, Morrow tendered his resignation. He practiced in Pittsburgh and Delphi, Indiana. (RLML)

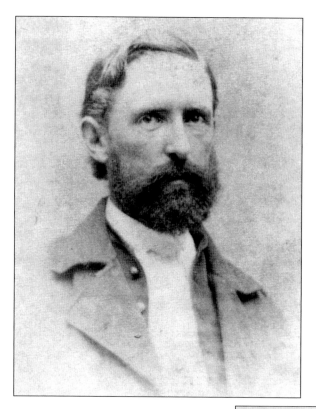

Dr. William Spencer of Monticello, Indiana, followed his father as assistant surgeon of the 73rd Indiana Infantry. His father died during his service. Spencer was captured and held for seven months in Libby Prison. After he was commissioned surgeon of the 10th Tennessee Cavalry, he wrote to Governor Morton, "I have been on the stool of repentance ever since I have been commissioned in the 10th Tennessee . . . I am mortified at serving out of the good old Hoosier State. Won't you take me back?" (Collection of John Sickles)

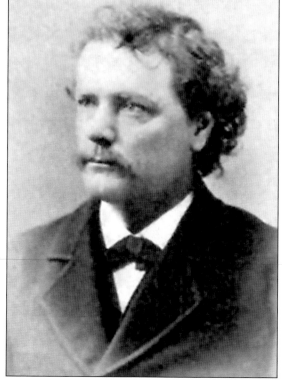

William Fletcher, a son of Calvin Fletcher of Indianapolis, served as a private for three months. In charge of secret service, he was captured and sentenced to hanging but was reprieved by General Lee. After parole, Fletcher began a hospital for Confederate prisoners in Indianapolis in a gymnasium at Meridian and Maryland Streets. He lectured about his experiences as a prisoner of the Confederates. The proceeds of these lectures went to Soldiers' Aid activities. (RLML)

Dr. Benjamin Newland had been an Indiana state senator for the Lawrence County District. His colonel wrote the following: "The 22nd Indiana from its organization to the present has suffered in the medical department through the following reasons: not wishing to perform the duties of Surgeon in the field or from other reason, some time after the organization of the Regiment B.F. Newland Surgeon of the Regiment through General Fremont was detailed as Post Surgeon at Jefferson City." (RLML)

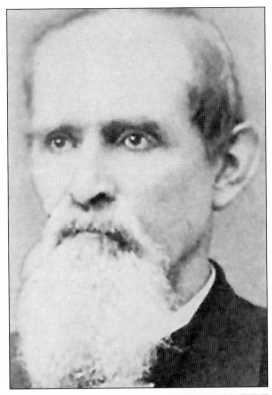

Benjamin Newland was a friend of General Jefferson C. Davis of Indiana. General Davis shot General William Nelson in the Galt House Hotel in Louisville in 1862. Dr. Newland was present and tended Nelson's fatal wounds. Davis never faced trial for the shooting. (HW)

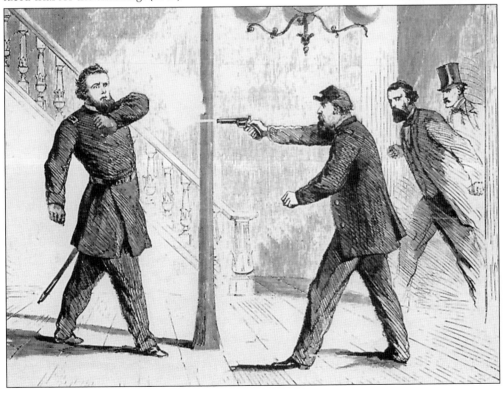

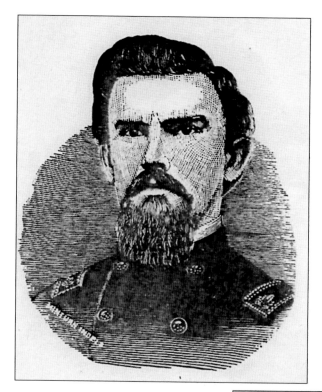

Dr. John P. Porter of Decatur, Indiana, surgeon of the 89th Indiana, died with Major Samuel Henry and other officers in Guntown near Lexington, Missouri. They stopped for dinner at a house in Guntown. As the end of their column passed, the woman cooking dinner remarked that rebel guerrillas in the area made it unsafe for them to remain there. However, Dr. Porter wanted more food. Guerrillas dressed as Union officers took Porter and the others prisoner and shot them. (RLML)

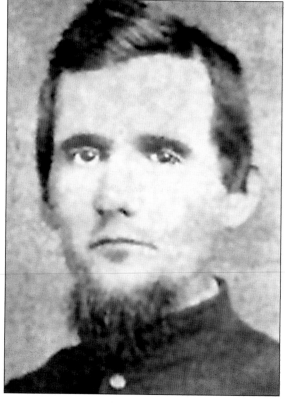

Isaac Casselberry of Evansville, Indiana, served with the 1st Indiana Cavalry. Ironically, he died of typhoid fever after the war. Typhoid fever was a common cause of death during the war. While Casselberry was medical director of General Steel's division, his horse was killed under him at the Battle of Mark's Mills, April 1864, and resulted in his capture and imprisonment for three months. He frequently conversed about military operations after the war. (RLML)

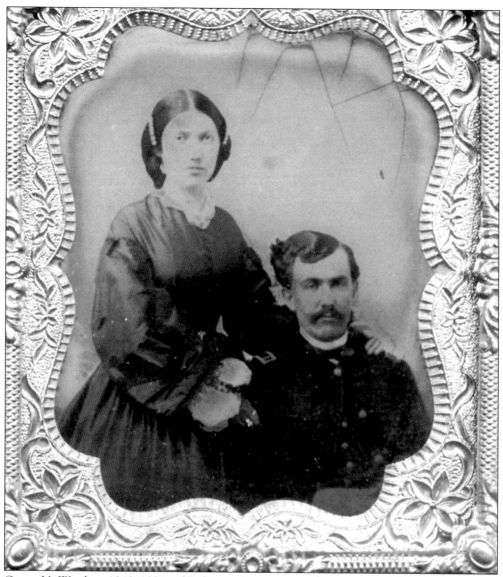

Green V. Woolen, 1840–1921, of Indianapolis was an assistant surgeon of the 27th Indiana. He spent many months as the surgeon in chief of the 12th Army Corps Artillery. After the war, he was in charge of City Hospital in Indianapolis (Wishard Memorial Hospital). He wrote a recollection that included a description of his captivity in Libby Prison. A woman nursing her sick husband was also captured. Woolen reported that the woman was raped and possibly murdered by the infamous Wirtz of Andersonville. It was reported that Drs. J.L. Thompson and G.V. Woolen of Indianapolis, "form a conspicuous and well known couple about the hotel headquarters of every American Medical Association meeting. Both were soldiers and surgeons in the Civil War." Woolen requested a leave in January 1864, to return to Indianapolis to visit his family and attend to urgent private business of a delicate nature pertaining to his family. Early in February 1864, he married Mary Smith of Indianapolis. After this leave, he was reassigned to the Murfreesboro hospital. (Courtesy of Richard Wyatt Brown)

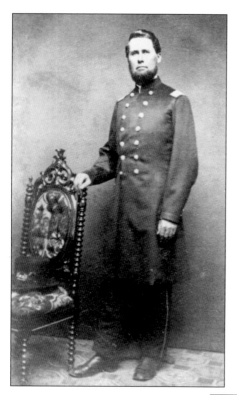

Dr. A.C. Fosdick of Liberty, Indiana, was additional surgeon protempore with the 36th Indiana Volunteers after Shiloh. Later he was commissioned as surgeon of the 5th Indiana Cavalry. The local newspaper said he was the picture of health and "Muchly Militaire." He soon had trouble requisitioning the necessary medical supplies. Like many other surgeons in volunteer regiments, Fosdick had trouble using the Army's medical forms and terminology. (Courtesy of the John Sickles Collection at USAMHI)

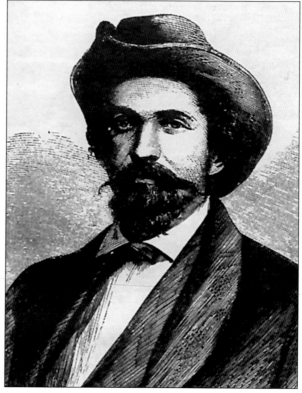

John Hunt Morgan and his band of Confederates raided Southern Indiana consistantly, stealing horses. Fosdick was present in Cincinnati when the captured officers of Morgan's command were being introduced to Federal officers. Dr. Fosdick declined the honor of an introduction, saying Morgan's men were horse thieves, and he would never accept the acquaintance of thieves. His controversial action made the Liberty newspapers. (RLML)

Dr. William Butterworth was commissioned as surgeon of the 99th. His letters to the *Mishawaka Enterprise* reveal a sense of humor and introspection. His attitude toward African Americans was humanized as he saw the struggle for freedom only began with the Emancipation Proclamation. Unfortunately, his diary was lost by a servant. Butterworth's grandson, Charles Butterworth, was a movie and stage star. (Regimental History.)

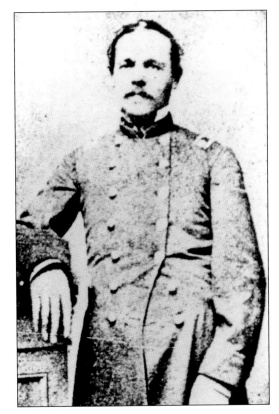

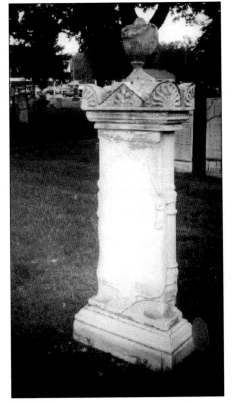

"Many graves are seen among these campgrounds. Often, as I pass over the knolls and sloping hill and see the little mounds and headboards that mark the fast, narrow homes of brave and loyal men, and think, how dear is this heart, and that, now cold in death around me, to homes in Indiana and Illinois, now shrouded in mourning, I ask if these men are to die in vain?"—William Butterworth. (Courtesy of Geneva McKenzie.)

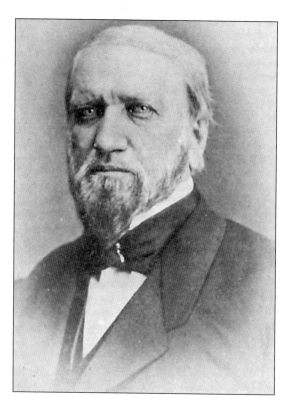

Ezra Read of Terre Haute was in the Army of the Republic of Texas as staff surgeon to General Felix Huston and on the Republic of Texas' ship, *Zavalla*. During the Civil War, he served in the 21st Indiana Infantry from Maryland to Louisiana, reporting on many diseases for the *Medical and Surgical History of the War of the Rebellion*. He eventually become a surgeon of the 11th Cavalry. (K)

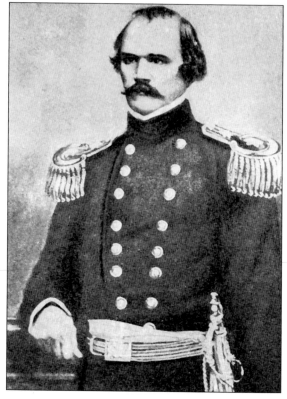

Albert Sidney Johnson, the future Confederate general, was wounded in a duel with Felix Huston during the war for Texas Independence. Ezra Read was one of the physicians who treated him. It is not known if Read was his surgeon at the location the injury was acquired or at Texana. Johnston's sciatic nerve was involved in the injury, and he later received a mortal wound at the battle of Shiloh. (RLML)

Six

Doctors
Good and Bad

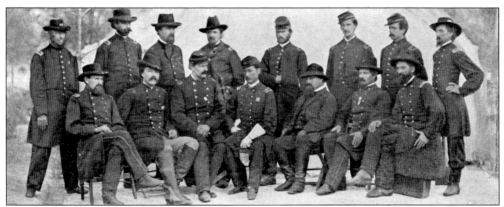

Many styles of hats are worn by this group of surgeons of 2nd Division 9th Corps. Likewise, the records of individual surgeons before, during, and after the war were not consistent. The confrontation between Drs. Bullard and Field that follows illustrates how two people with good intentions can see a situation in two completely different ways. Military discipline was unknown to these physicians and inexperienced volunteer officers were unaware of the importance of camp hygiene and rest for ailing soldiers. (MPH)

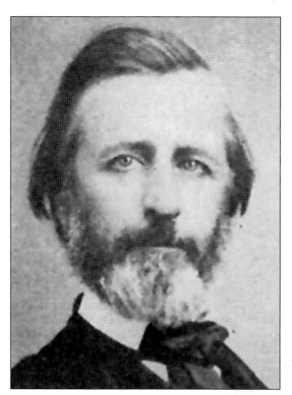

Talbott Bullard, brother-in-law of Henry Ward Beecher, organized a hospital for the sick Confederate prisoners at the Old Post Office Building, and examined recruits in Indianapolis. He made a trip for Governor Morton to the battlefields of Richmond, Kentucky. During this trip, his party of doctors and nurses was greeted by Dr. N. Field in a less than gracious manner. On a trip to Vicksburg, Bullard contracted a fatal disease. (RLML)

Dr. Nathaniel Field of the 66th Indiana Infantry responded to Bullard's criticism of his hospital. He published affidavits from a local Richmond, Kentucky, minister who stayed at the Madison Female Seminary as wound dresser. He testified that over 350 men were in the house when Field came to the hospital. The minister affirmed that the house smelled but what else could be expected when 300 wounded and over 1,000 prisoners had been housed on the grounds. (RLML)

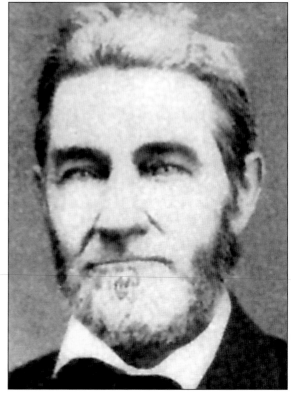

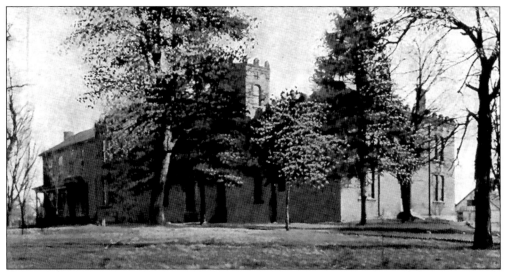

At the Madison Seminary, Dr. Field was dependent on the Confederates and the benevolence of the citizens for supplies. The minister testified that it was impossible to procure water and that the yard was getting to be a privy on a large scale. Dr. Bullard arrived with a large party including many women and expected Dr. Field to provide them with appropriate lodging and was horrified with the odors. (Courtesy of Eastern Kentucky University Special Collections)

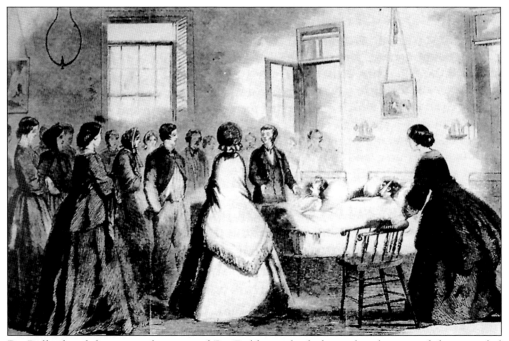

Dr. Bullard with his party of nurses and Dr. Field were both doing their best to aid the wounded after the Battle of Richmond. The minister declared in defense of Dr. Field, "I do believe that any person could possibly have done better under all the circumstances than did Dr. Field after he was appointed post Surgeon of the Seminary Hospital." Impossible circumstances frequently thwarted the best efforts of surgeons. (RLML)

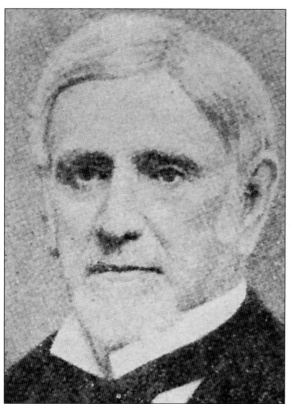

Patrick Henry Jameson of Indianapolis was put in charge of "everything" medical for soldiers not yet assigned to regiments. He was also in charge of Confederate prisoners captured at Ft. Donelson at Camp Morton. He sat in a buggy and watched them leave when they were exchanged and freed. He claimed not to have missed a day of duty in five years. (RLML)

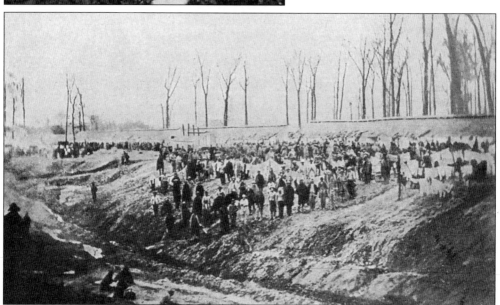

Camp Morton in Indianapolis housed up to 4,999 Confederate prisoners at one time. Confederate prisoners were hospitalized in several buildings in downtown Indianapolis beside the City Hospital. Confederate surgeons among the prisoners, as well as captured African-American slaves, helped to care for them. At one point, the doctors in charge were ordered to remove Union soldiers from City Hospital to make room for ill Confederates. (MPH)

Orpheus Everts was surgeon of the 20th Indiana and a brigade surgeon in the Army of the Potomac missing only the First Battle of Bull Run and Antietam. He took courses at the Medical College of Indiana (LaPorte) and was later editor of *The Laporte Times*, a pro-slavery Democratic newspaper. After the war, he furthered his medical studies specializing in diseases of the nervous system, a field later identified with psychiatry. (K)

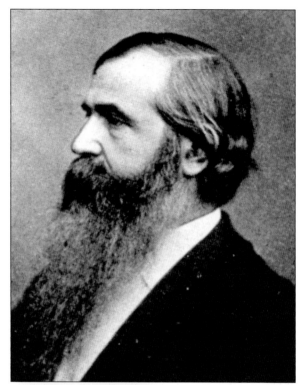

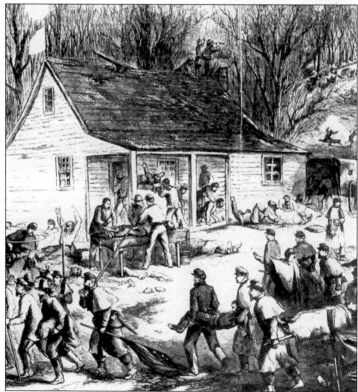

S.T. Montgomery described Everts during the Battle of Fredericksburg: "Medical Director, Dr. Everts, was every where present: thus encouraging the entire Medical force to the use of every means possible for the alleviation of human suffering . . . and I never shall forget the experience of the four days thus engaged. Men mangled in every conceivable place were provided for and I tell you that the human suffering was terrible." (HW)

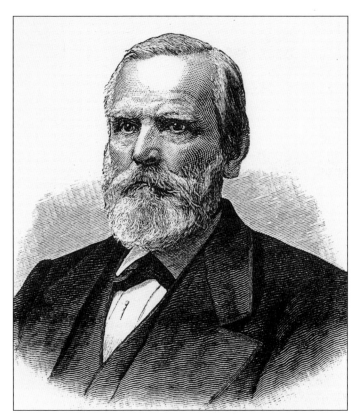

Surgeon George Washington New of Indianapolis, surgeon of the 7th Indiana Infantry, was court-martialed for selling whisky and brandy to the soldiers. He claimed there was no way to move it. He was reinstated probably by Governor Morton. Surgeon New had entered the service bringing with him his wife and son. After his reinstatement, he was brigade and corps surgeon. New was also one of Governor Morton's military agents in New Orleans. (RLML)

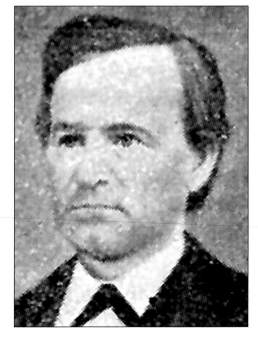

Alexander M. Murphy and son Alexander Dudley Murphy of Sullivan served with the 97th Indiana and were well-liked. The senior Murphy was reported to be an excellent man and a good surgeon ready with both medicines for the sick and care for the wounded, as well as with words of comfort and sympathy. Although "Dud" was popular with his regiment, he was reported to have been in the company of a young woman at the end of a drinking spree spanning several days when he died. (RLML)

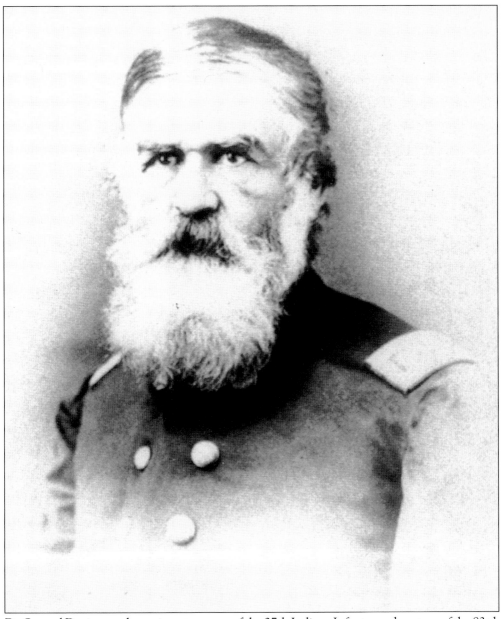

Dr. Samuel Davis served as assistant surgeon of the 37th Indiana Infantry and surgeon of the 83rd. His record makes it plain he was dedicated to the Abolitionist cause. Born in Ontario County, New York, he studied at Oberlin College, the first institution to admit African Americans. He went to Cincinnati in 1834 where he taught at a school for African Americans while attending medical school, and was a participant in the publication of the Abolitionist newspaper, *Philanthropist*. In 1838, he moved to Franklin County, Indiana, and was elected to the Indiana House and served from 1851 to 1852. His regimental history relates that he had over 300 sick to care for at Young's Point, caring not only for those in his own regiment but for the 69th as well. He was praised for his untiring will as the regiments labored to construct a canal. He later fell from an ambulance, causing a permanent spine injury. (Courtesy of civilwarindiana.com)

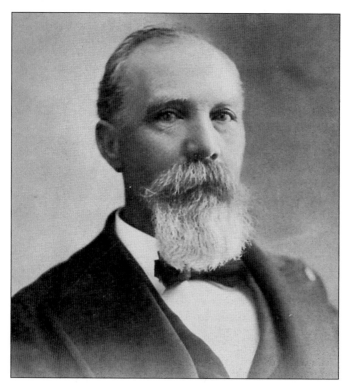

Of John S. McPheeters of the 23rd Indiana Infantry, an Iowa surgeon said, " I find him skillful, industrious, energetic and faithful, understanding his business and doing his duty well and promptly." McPheeters wanted to resign. His colonel wrote him, begging him to stay: "If you and Brucker both leave some damned quack will be shoved in on us as has been the case always until yourself and Brucker came." McPheeters was General Nathan Kimball's nephew and lived in Washington County, Indiana. (RLML)

George Malin Collins, 1838–1896, did not graduate from Cincinnati College of Medicine and Surgery until 1863. In 1864, he was appointed assistant surgeon of the 17th Indiana Regiment. Collins had studied with the surgeon of the 17th, J.Y. Hitt. He practiced in Rush, Shelby, and Tipton Counties in Indiana. (Courtesy of the Indiana State Library, Manuscript Section, Picture Collection)

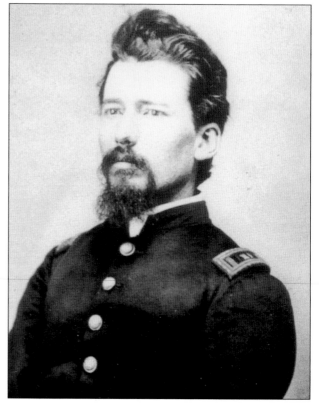

John F. Taggart of Clark County, Indiana served in the 4th Cavalry. One person who saw his hospital in Cairo, Illinois, said he could not do it justice for it was the best hospital between there and New Orleans. Mary Livermore called Taggart "one of the noblest of men put in his place." Taggart was known to be kind-hearted, careful, and skillful. (Courtesy of civilwarindiana.com)

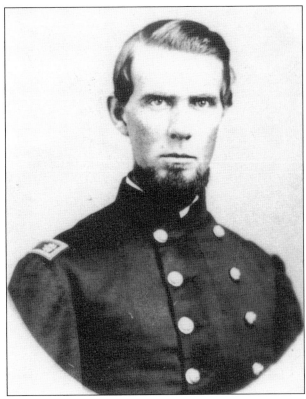

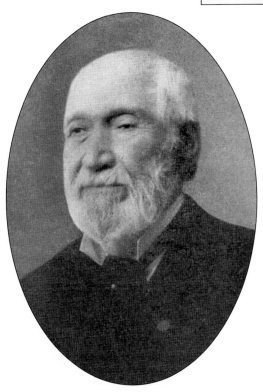

William Boor, the surgeon of the 4th Indiana Cavalry, was appointed Brigade Surgeon of the Army of the Cumberland. He practiced 11 years in Middletown, Indiana. There he led efforts to ban intoxicants. His second wife Sarah A.R. Roof took over her husband's business interests in New Castle during the war. She sent him monthly and quarterly statements. Mrs. Boor may have been the only surgeon's wife who was for women's suffrage. (K)

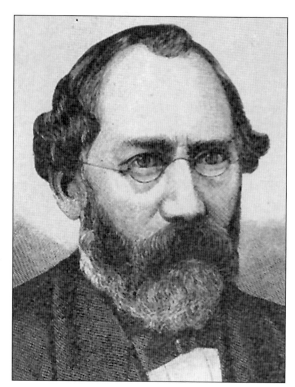

Alois D. Gall of Indianapolis was born in Wiel die Stadt, Wurtemberg, Germany. He was U.S. Consul to Antwerp for six years before the Civil War. As surgeon of the 13th, he was in charge in the Female Seminary Hospital at Winchester, Virginia, and later Medical Director of General Peck's Corps. He received a sword for his service from his fellow officers. (RLML)

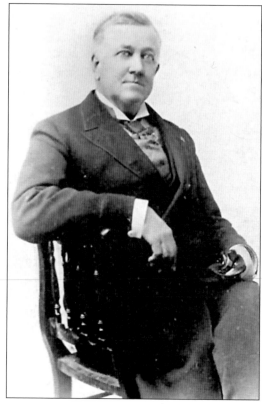

James J. Rooker of Castleton, Indiana was a founder of the Central College of Physicians and Surgeons in Indianapolis, along with several other former regimental surgeons. Rooker's official request to resign contains this comment from the Lt. Colonel of the 11th: "I beg that this worse than useless officer be allowed to leave the service. His resignation is the first real benefit to the service has ever received." (RLML)

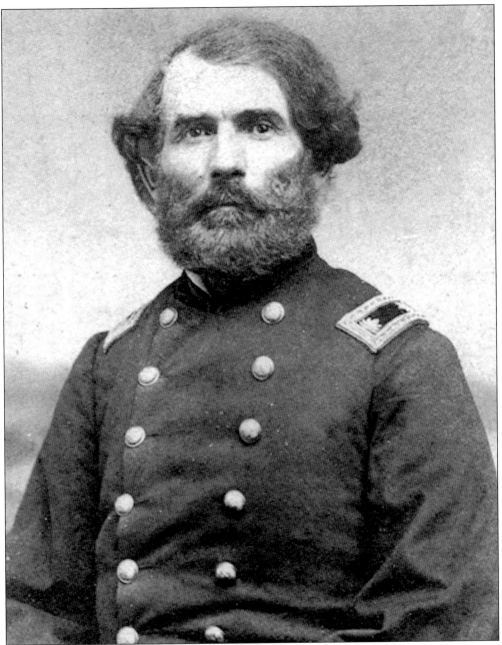

Caleb V. Jones was born in New York in 1812. He came to Indiana in 1838, serving in the state senate from 1843 to 1846 for Fountain County. He was surgeon for the 1st Indiana Regiment during the Mexican War, and was a special assistant surgeon appointed by the governor of the 40th Indiana from 1862 to 1863, and later was surgeon of the 73rd from 1863 to 1864. His obituary states that many soldiers recount his acts of kindness, including giving up his horse for the tired soldiers to ride. Immediately following the war, Jones became the first president of the Fountain County Medical Society. However, he received a court martial for conduct unbecoming an officer. He "cursed and abused a sick private" and using language unbecoming an officer, he "called the colonel a damned little whiffet." (Courtesy of <u>civilwarindiana.com</u>)

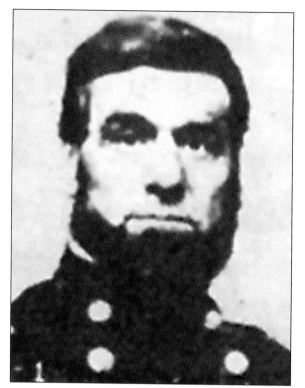

Daniel Meeker, 9th Indiana, was professor of Surgery at Indiana Medical College at LaPorte, Indiana. He was the father of the Mayo Brothers. His students knew him as "Doctor Death," an appellation we hope was unknown to his patients. Later in life, Dr. Meeker advertised Dr. Meeker's Opium Cure. Advertising a secret cure resulted in his ejection from the Indiana State Medical Society, of which he had been the president. (RLML)

In early 1863, Sylvester Laning of North Liberty, Indiana, an assistant surgeon of the 48th Indiana, wrote home concerning the feelings of soldiers in regard to the Emancipation Proclamation. A Democrat, Laning wrote that the Proclamation made no difference, since slavery in fact ceased to exist wherever the Union Army went. After the war, he left North Liberty and settled in Kingman, Kansas. By proclamation of the mayor of Kingman, all businesses closed for his funeral. (Courtesy of the Indiana State Library Manuscript Section, Picture Collection)

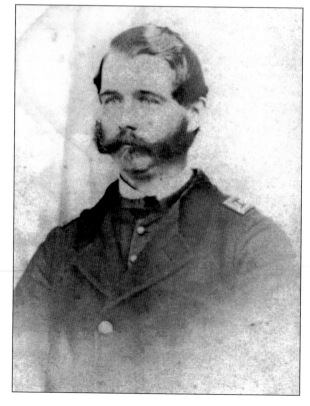

James Walter Hervey of Hancock County, an assistant surgeon of the 50th Indiana, was injured when a hospital fell on him near Parker's Cross Roads, Tennessee. In 1858 he wrote a horror and temperance novel, *The Scroll and the Locket; or the Maniac of the Mound.* "Oh rum, we hate thee! Thou hast wronged us much! Thou hast scattered our friends and heaped sorrow upon our heart. Our mind is overburdened with the memory of thy rule." (RLML)

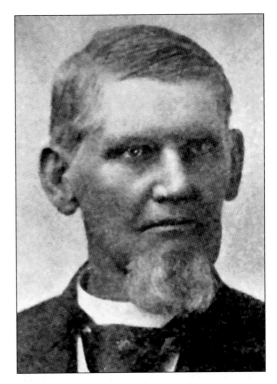

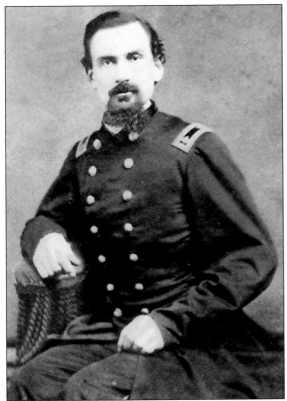

Joshua Whittington Underhill of the 46th Indiana Infantry served well and kept a diary. He lost the diary at Vicksburg, but miraculously it was returned to him months later. While he maintained a respectable medical career in Cincinnati, the hard working Dr. Underhill experimented with cocaine and died a victim of his addiction. Several prominent American doctors also fell victim to this new drug. (Courtesy of Philip Morss)

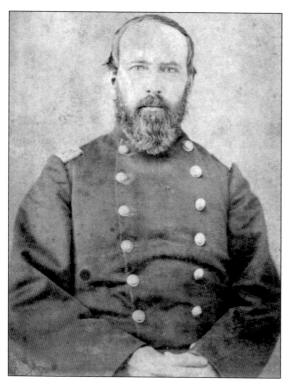

Wilson Hobbs practiced for many years in Knightstown, Indiana. Born in Salem, Indiana, he lost his mother to complications after childbirth and his father to cholera. His family was a member of the Society of Friends, and Hobbs is one of several surgeons with Quaker connections. He attended the University of Michigan, and set up practice in Annapolis, Indiana. Hobbs was a commissioned surgeon of the 85th regiment. One officer writes home, "No finer man ever wielded a scalpel. His kindness to the sick on their lonely couches of pain, has won for him the most sincere friendship of this regiment; much more than can be said of most surgeons in the army. I have yet to hear of his ever compelling a man to march when the man said he was unable to do so. No air, the 85th can't spare Dr. Hobbs." He was brigade surgeon of the 1st Brigade, Second Division, Cavalry Corps of the Army of the Cumberland. He was later president of the Indiana State Medical Society. (Courtesy of civilwarindiana.com)

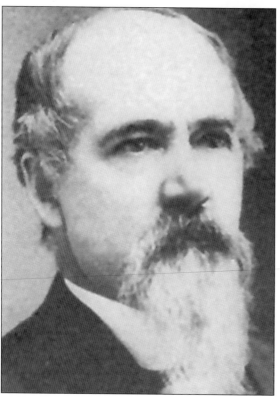

Seven

AFTER THE WAR

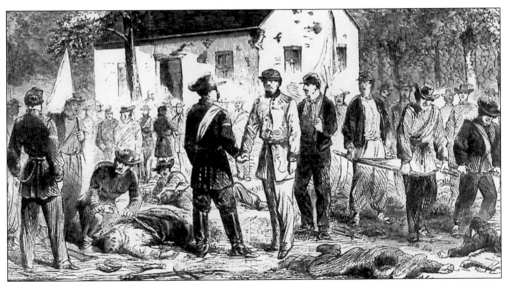

Flags of truce allowed doctors to find and treat patients in the hands of the enemy. Like the officers who attended West Point, doctors had often been classmates at medical school before they faced each other on the battlefield. After the war, physicians of the American Medical Society were quick to re-unite the profession. Former Confederate surgeons did form their own medical society but the elite, as before, participated in the American Medical Association. The AMA symbolically held its 1869 meeting in New Orleans. The medical profession took many steps towards professionalization often lead by former Civil War surgeons. (HW)

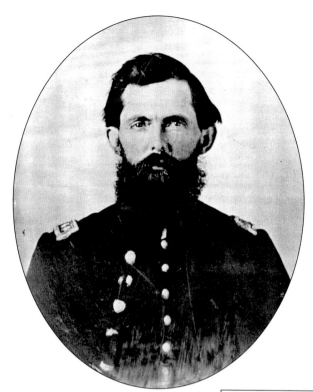

Samuel Tyner was born and practiced in Warrick County. He was a member of Co. K, 42nd Regiment of which he became surgeon. He returned home and began to plow his fields. After only an hour or two, he ran into a hornet's nest, which made the horses bolt. The plow was destroyed and the harness ruined. He discussed the situation with his wife and entered Rush Medical College of Chicago immediately. (Courtesy of civilwarindiana.com)

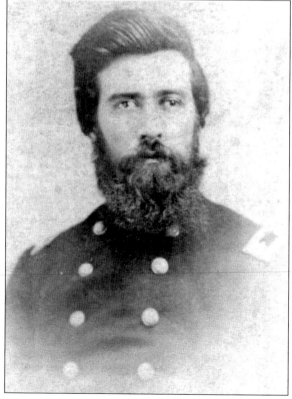

The pension record of Dr. Francis Pearman of Kosciusko County is typical. He claimed to have been disabled with heart disease and chronic diarrhea acquired in the army. The chronic diarrhea of veterans was probably dysentery they acquired from drinking contaminated water during the war. The pensions were usually awarded at some level. (Courtesy of the Indiana State Library, Manuscript Section, Picture Collection)

William Freeman lived the stereotype of the drunken surgeon while serving with the 7th Indiana Cavalry. His military records indicate that in a drunken rage he vowed to kill the regiment's Colonel Shanks. Shanks disarmed Freeman, who was dismissed from service May 10, 1864. Freeman was later in life appointed president of the Jay County Medical Society. Ironically, his obituary specifically refers to his service with Colonel Shanks. (Courtesy of John Sickles)

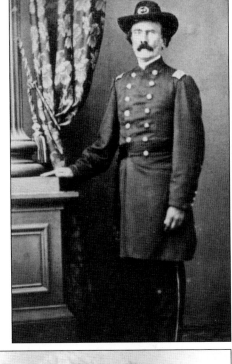

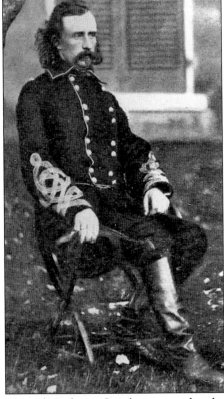

The 7th Indiana Cavalry was under the command of General George Armstrong Custer. The regimental historian called him a person of unusual egotism and self-importance as well as a fop and a dandy. Further, he shot deserters without referring the matter to the president. (MPH)

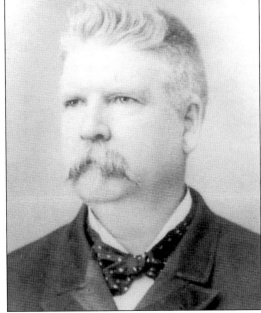

Dr. Chitwood of Connersville was one of the special surgeons appointed by Governor Morton to Shiloh as an additional surgeon. Joshua Chitwood of Connersville was Surgeon of the 7th Indiana Cavalry and was then promoted to surgeon in chief of the 7th Cavalry Division. He was later on the staff of General Custer. (RLML)

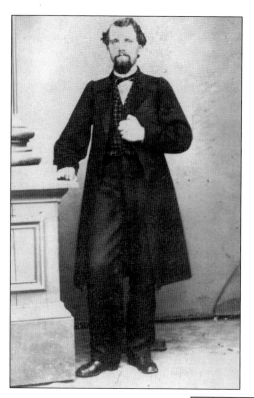

Charles Abbett of Muncie, Indiana, served as an assistant surgeon of the 36th regiment. This photo shows him in civilian dress, illustrating how a doctor from a large Indiana town might have dressed around the time of the Civil War. The financial status of a physician often had more to do with his family's financial status than the success of his practice. Physicians frequently supplemented the proceeds of their profession with land dealing, farming, or other businesses. (Courtesy of civilwarindiana.com)

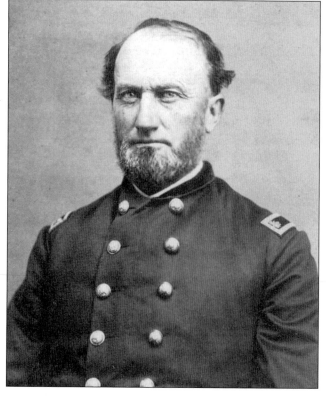

Vincent Gregg, 1825–1895, came to Connersville in 1858. As did many other surgeons, he went to Shiloh as a volunteer. He was made surgeon of the 124th Indiana and was made surgeon of the 1st Brigade, 1st Division of the 23rd Army Corps. Later, hospitals in Charlotte and Greensborough, North Carolina, were in his charge. (Courtesy of Richard Wyman Brown.)

Dr. Lewis Humphreys served with the 29th Indiana and was the second mayor of South Bend. He was placed in a similar position of leadership during the war as medical inspector. Medical inspectors provided a link between the few leaders of the regular army at the top and the thousands of regimental and volunteer surgeons. He completed his service in the St. Louis area. (Photo courtesy of civilwarindiana.com)

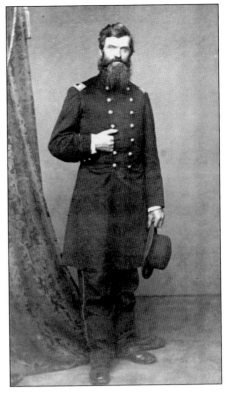

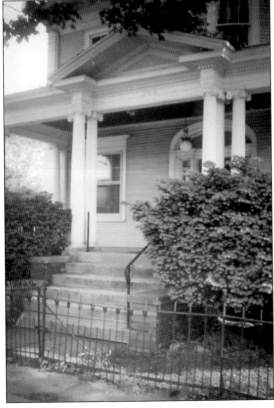

Dr. Humphreys was a prime example of a successful physician. His home built after the Civil War was typical of physicians' homes in cities. Doctors often had their offices in their homes or saw patients both at home and at the office. Their ads often gave the office and home location. (Courtesy of Geneva McKenzie)

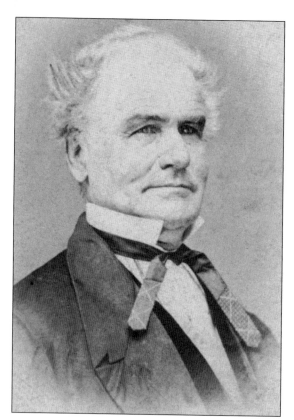

Levi Ham of the 48th Indiana was a native of Maine. He practiced medicine, was a state senator, and was superintendent of the Maine Asylum for the Insane. He moved to New York and then to South Bend in 1859. He was appointed surgeon of the 48th Indiana and was soon put in charge of one of the hospitals in Paducah, Kentucky, filled with wounded from Fort Donelson and Shiloh. He was reported to have operated for nearly 8 days straight. He asked to rejoin his regiment and became chairman of the operating board of the 7th Division of the 17th Corps. At 60 years of age he was Medical Director of the 17th Corps under General McPherson. In 1880, Dr. Ham became the first Democrat to be elected mayor of South Bend. (Courtesy of Northern Indiana Center for History Archives)

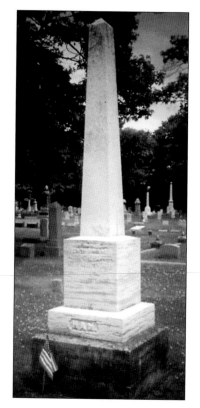

Pictured here is the tombstone for the Ham family. (Courtesy of Geneva McKenzie)

Entering the 9th Indiana Cavalry as private, Edwin W. Magann was hospital steward and later assistant surgeon. Enlisting late in 1863, he was taken prisoner at Sulphur Trestle, Alabama, in 1864. He suffered a dislocated shoulder and spinal contusions. The doctor became a patient in the Nashville Officers' Hospital and a convalescent hospital in Louisville. Records do not show any indication that he was ever a practicing physician. (Courtesy of John Sickles)

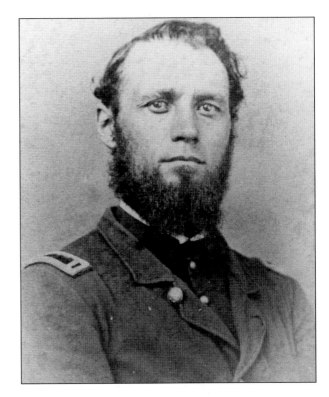

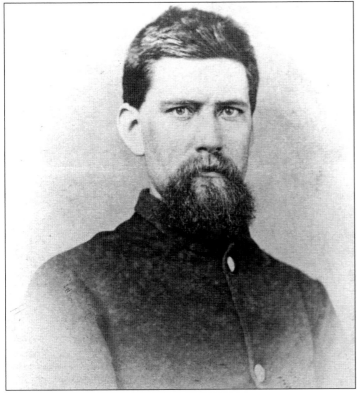

Young Thomas J. Adams had studied medicine in Hendricks County and was teaching school when he enlisted in the 9th Indiana Cavalry. Appointed hospital steward, he served during the Battles at Columbia, Franklin, and Nashville. After Nashville, Steward Adams gathered up many wounded and placed them on the ambulances, and after the war, attended medical school. (Courtesy of John Sickles)

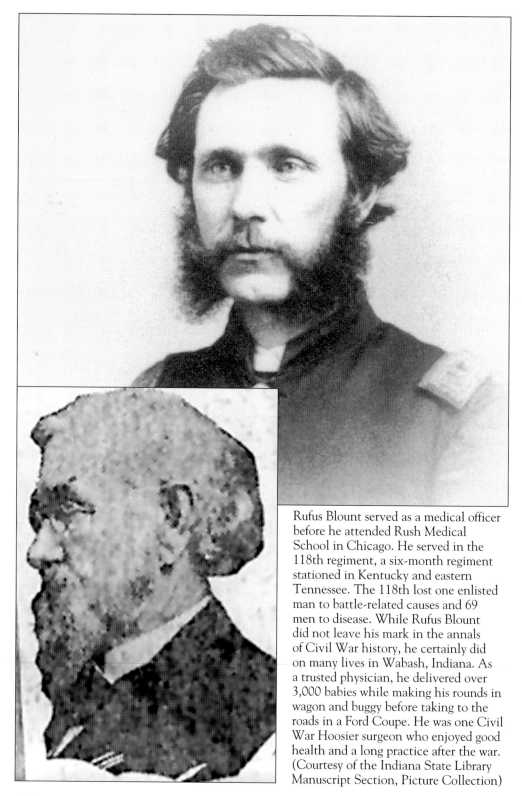

Rufus Blount served as a medical officer before he attended Rush Medical School in Chicago. He served in the 118th regiment, a six-month regiment stationed in Kentucky and eastern Tennessee. The 118th lost one enlisted man to battle-related causes and 69 men to disease. While Rufus Blount did not leave his mark in the annals of Civil War history, he certainly did on many lives in Wabash, Indiana. As a trusted physician, he delivered over 3,000 babies while making his rounds in wagon and buggy before taking to the roads in a Ford Coupe. He was one Civil War Hoosier surgeon who enjoyed good health and a long practice after the war. (Courtesy of the Indiana State Library Manuscript Section, Picture Collection)

The pension records of
John H. Ford, 93rd Indiana
Infantry, indicate he was either
consumptive before he entered
the service or contracted
tuberculosis soon after joining
the army. Marion Mooney of
Columbus, Indiana, 1st Lt. of
Co. E 93rd stated, "We had
a mutual dislike one for the
other and I ordered him to
the front but he in a few days
with the necessary written
orders returned and assumed
medical charge. He was then
sick as I could see and suffered
much from this."(Courtesy of
USAMHI and John Sickles)

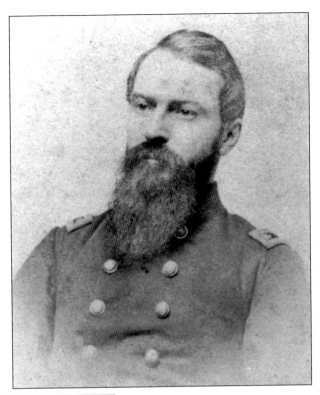

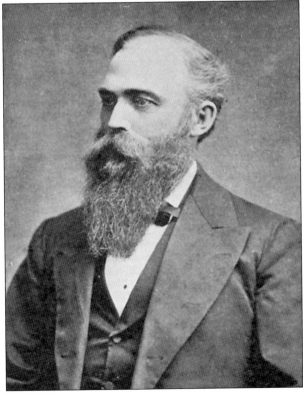

Flavius Josephus VanVorhis,
1841–1913, was a native of
Marion County Indiana. He
was an assistant surgeon of the
86th regiment. He, as did many
other Civil War surgeons, took
great interest in public health
after the war. VanVorhis was
known as the father of health
legislation in Indiana. (RLML)

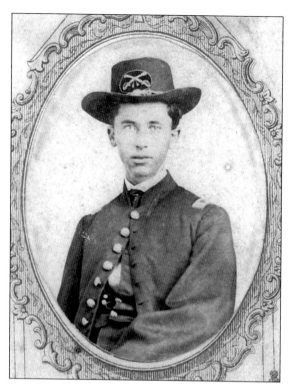

Robert Harrison Crowder of Sullivan, Indiana, a former school teacher and student at Rush Medical College, married in 1861. In 1863 he became the captain of Co. G., 11th Indiana Cavalry and surgeon of the regiment. Crowder was at various times in the grocery, drug, and real estate business in Sullivan. All this time he continued serving the town as a physician, making the rigorous house calls required during that time. (Courtesy of John Croff).

James Tolerton lived in Whitely and Fulton County. He was surgeon of 129th Indiana. The 129th participated in the Siege of Atlanta and the Battles Franklin and Nashville. Although the regiment was not mustered until early 1864, it lost 19 men to mortal injuries and 166 to disease. (Courtesy of Mark Weldon.)

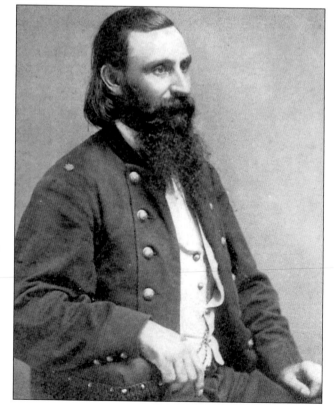

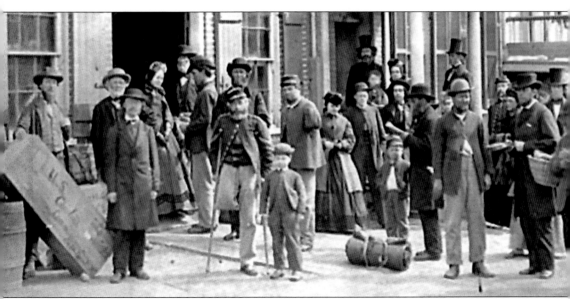

After the war, wounded, ill, and healthy veterans alike formed a powerful voting block in post-war America. Veteran's hospitals and homes appeared in parts of the U.S. The Grand Army of the Republic (G.A.R) veterans group lobbied for higher pensions and secured political patronage jobs for veterans. Local G.A.R. posts were often named for fallen local heroes, including one named for Dr. Thomas W.C. Williamson of the 24th Indiana of Paoli. Williamson was killed at the Battle of Champion Hill while attending to a soldier struck in the leg with a mini-ball. Dr. Williamson was cutting it out when he received his fatal wound. (MPH)

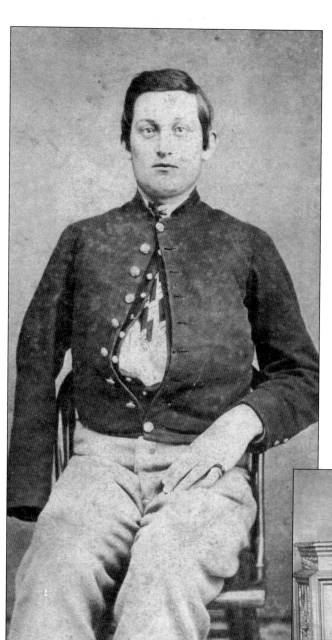

James Thomas (1845–1914) of the 57th Indiana was typical of many young Hoosier farmers who served in the Civil War. When he was 19 years old, he was wounded at Kennesaw Mountain, Georgia. His wound required Dr. W.B. McGavron of the 26th Ohio Infantry to amputate his right arm by the flap method. This meant that skin was folded over the remaining limb forming a natural covering of the stump. Movies and novels give the impression that young Thomas pined away a helpless cripple. The amputation was far from the end of Thomas' life. He avoided contracting gangrene, went home, married in 1865, fathered seven children and owned a hardware store in Greenfield, Indiana. He was the county recorder for eight years and commander of the Samuel Dunbar G.A.R., Grand Army of the Republic, post. (Courtesy of John Sickles)

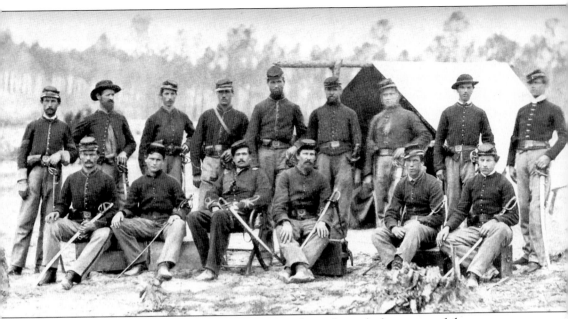

"Many of the survivors of the war are far greater physical wrecks by reason of the exposures and sickness of the camp and march, than those are who lost limbs in battle. The Adjutant-General of Indiana in his Official Report of the troops from our State, very properly and justly places the men, who died of diseases, side by side in the roll of honor with those who fell in battle. Men dying in hospitals, away from home, unattended by their friends, 'paid the last full measure of their devotion,' as truly as those who were shot down on the battlefield. They died to secure a Union victory just as much as they would have done in a charging column." This passage is from the history of the 57th Regiment. The photograph is of men of the 3rd Indiana Cavalry. (MPH)

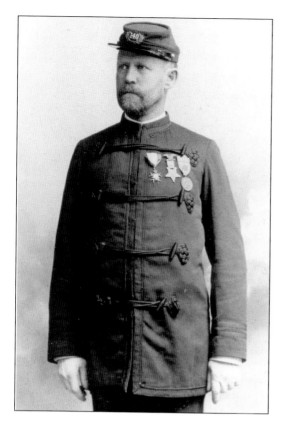

William H. Lemon of Clay and Monroe Counties, Indiana, was assistant and surgeon of the 82nd Indiana. Here he wears the uniform of the 140th G.A.R. post in New York. His death was recorded to have occurred in Lawrence, Kansas. One of his children was born in Iowa, one in Illinois, and two in Indiana.(Courtesy of USAMHI)

William Cole of Fountain County, surgeon of the 6th Cavalry, was a veteran of the regular army during the Mexican War. He is reported to have graduated from the Medical College of Ohio. He participated in the Fountain County Medical Society, Indiana State Medical Society, the American Medical Society, and attended a medical congress in Mexico City in 1892. (Courtesy of John Sickles)

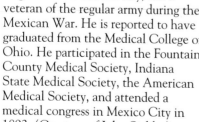

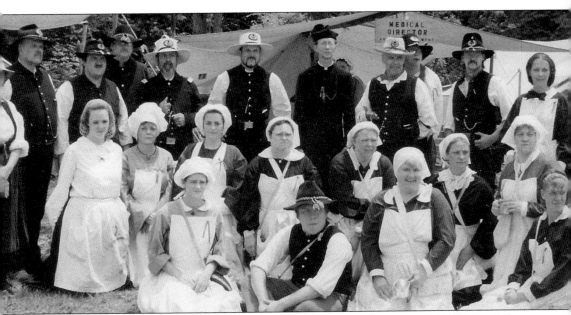

The work of Civil War surgeons is preserved by Civil War medical reenactors. In 1992 at Billie Creek Village near Rockville, Indiana, a large gathering of Civil War medical reenactors took place. This group includes them portraying nurses and surgeons. Two groups devote their full time to the study of Civil War medicine: the Society of Civil War Surgeons and the National Museum of Civil War Medicine. (Courtesy of Peter J. D'Onofrio)

Index